Critiquing Nursing Research

Note

Health care practice and knowledge are constantly changing and developing as new research and treatments, changes in procedures, drugs and equipment become available.

The author and publishers have, as far as is possible, taken care to confirm that the information complies with the latest standards of practice and legislation.

Critiquing Nursing Research

2nd edition

John Cutcliffe and Martin Ward

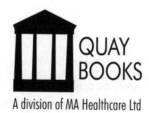

QUAY
BOOKS

A division of MA Healthcare Ltd

Quay Books Division, MA Healthcare Ltd, St Jude's Church, Dulwich Road, London SE24 0PB

British Library Cataloguing-in-Publication Data
A catalogue record is available for this book

© MA Healthcare Limited 2007

ISBN-13: 987 1 85642 316 8
ISBN-10: 1 85642 316 6

Printed by Ashford Colour Press Ltd, Gosport, Hants, PO13 0FW

Contents

Foreword to the first edition

The Royal College of Nursing Institute is proud to have been associated with the establishment of the Network for Psychiatric Nursing Research (NPNR) in the mid-1990s. As host for this Department of Health (England) funded innovation, the spirit and commitment shown by the originators of the idea, were very much in synchrony with the aspirations and vision of the Institute.

The authors of this book have provided us with a detailed outline of how the network developed, what it was trying to achieve and how it has refined its purposes. Responding to the policy imperative of the evidence-based practice movement, the founders of NPNR have been able to combine the essential ingredients of effective utilisation of evidence into practice; namely, the ability to critique research with a practitioner/researcher network of interested, committed individuals. This combination of critical appraisal skill development (covering both conventional quantitative and qualitative approaches) with dissemination and networking strategies is still quite a rare phenomenon. And the efforts of all those volunteers, who have contributed their intellectual and clinical expertise by way of being involved in critiquing research, or attending NPNR conferences, should also be acknowledged.

But the last words rightly rest with the authors themselves on the future direction of this timely and important initiative. Acknowledging the changing policy and practice landscape, the evolution of a much more integrated, interprofessional, person-centred research agenda and the impact of technology on research dissemination and implementation methods, Cutcliffe and Ward comment:

> ... Our future success lies in combining all the evidence resources at our disposal, including research, with the spontaneity of our intuitive actions and subjecting both to the same level of critical evaluation. In short, raising the level of our professional thinking to a more mature status.

This book offers one perspective on this journey.

Alison Kitson RN, PhD, FRCN
Executive Director, Nursing
Royal College of Nursing
April 2003

Foreword to the second edition

Apart from the genuine sense of honour that I experienced when I was asked to write the foreword for this book, I also felt that the invitation was timely for another reason. As I write this foreword, I am in the process of retiring from my post at the Institute of Psychiatry, King's College London, where I have held a Chair of Psychiatric Nursing since 1995. Such an occasion obviously prompts one to look back over one's career and to consider the way in which knowledge has evolved. As I read the manuscript for this book, I observed that John Cutcliffe and Martin Ward were, in their own way, engaged in a very similar process. That there is now a second edition of this book testifies to the way that our thinking about nursing research has evolved. For my part, I mistakenly thought at the time that I completed my PhD in the early 1980s that the then embryonic movement towards evidence-based medicine in psychiatry would have very clear-cut and positive results for nursing research. As it transpired, the evidence-based approach has brought major benefits – not only to research, but also to patient care. However, at the same time our understanding of what constitutes evidence is, in some senses, less clear now than it was a decade ago. We have come to realise that, although the randomised controlled trial is the gold standard for evaluating the outcomes of treatment, in mental health care the majority of studies published in journals are, from a statistical point of view, grossly under-powered, and many of the measures that we use are riddled with imperfections. If we set these problems alongside the way that we have now developed more robust methods in qualitative research, and the need to justify everything in terms of cost, we have a research scenario that defies simple description. We also need to note that, in mental health care particularly, while evidence, efficacy and effectiveness now constitute imperatives for all services delivering care and treatment, implementation of our knowledge is another matter. We now know that mental health care is beset by a range of problems in implementation, including fidelity to model, the lack of training capacity, and, once more, the issue of cost.

The rationale for the first edition of this book was based on the increasing need for nurses not only to become conversant with research, but also to consider evidence with a critical eye. This rationale is even more pertinent today than at the time of writing the first edition. The book provides nurses, in both the research and clinical fields, with a considerable resource in terms of understanding and critiquing, and this – of course – should have beneficial consequences for patient care. John Cutcliffe and Martin Ward have added to the first edition, which at the time was both comprehensive and authoritative, new material that will be of tremendous assistance to research students in their 'writing up', and have also put their original work into the European and broader global context.

I have no doubt that this is a book that will reach researchers at all levels. It will provide the undergraduate with a very useful template; assist the clinical nurse who will be faced with conflicting opinions about what is best for patient care; be a tremendous resource for those writing up research; and, finally, for those who consider themselves senior in the research field, might serve as a wake-up call.

One piece of advice I give frequently, particularly to those working in the field of evidence based medicine, is: 'To know what you don't know'. One might also add the advice: 'If you do know – what is the basis for your knowing and how sound is that basis?'. This book certainly provides an additional instrument in the toolkit of anyone who is setting out to look at knowledge and its acquisition. I look forward to the inevitable third edition, written in years to come, when those things we are certain about today are under scrutiny once more.

Kevin Gournay CBE
FRCPsych (Hon) FMedSci FRCN CPsychol AFBPsS RN PhD DSc
Emeritus Professor, Institute of Psychiatry, King's College London
July 2006

Preface to the first edition

The reasons for writing this book are best summarised under three points:

- There is a distinct absence of books that focus specifically on critiquing nursing research.
- There is an increasing requirement for nurses to become conversant with research, understand its link with the use of evidence to underpin practice and move towards being a evidence-based discipline.
- A crucial aspect of this increased 'mindfulness' of research is an awareness of the contemporary research issues facing nursing and the wider policy, multidisciplinary and political contexts in which these issues are embedded.

Consequently, we feel that having read this book readers should gain an appropriate knowledge and awareness pertaining to these three points. Nurses should be more familiar with some of the approaches and techniques involved in critiquing nursing research and be able to utilise some of these skills and techniques in their own efforts to critique. Accordingly, they will be better placed to make informed judgements regarding the quality of the research paper and the value of the evidence reported. Finally, they should also be able to locate the critiqued paper(s) within the wider policy, multidisciplinary and political contexts.

The book is divided into four integrated parts.

- Part 1 contains chapters which set the context and background to critiquing nursing research, explain the purpose and value of the critiquing process and describe the evolution of the Network for Psychiatric Nursing Research (NPNR) and its National Journal Club.
- Part 2 is comprised of a range of approaches used to critique nursing research and identifies the strengths and limitations of these approaches. Each approach is also accompanied by two examples of critiques, which are based on critiques undertaken by the NPNR National Journal Club.
- In Part 3, the NPNR National Journal Club's approach to critiquing nursing research is described. Since this is a developmental approach, we provide two additional examples for each of the four stages identified (a total of 16 different critiques of nursing research papers are included throughout the book).

■ The final part contains a chapter which discusses contemporary trends and themes in psychiatric/mental health nursing research and considers the complex relationship between psychiatric/mental health nursing research and multidisciplinary, collaborative research in the formal area of 'psychiatric care'. It also looks at the responsibilities for research of both nurse researchers and non-researchers.

The reader will notice that the papers reviewed using the NPNR National Journal Club approach are presented after the reviews undertaken using a range of models. This sequence of reviews was carried out purposefully in this 'order' since we wanted an approach to evolve and develop out of the National Journal Club work. Having done so, we were able to compare and contrast our approach with this range of approaches.

John R. Cutcliffe and Martin F. Ward
November 2002

Preface to the second edition

The authors of this book are delighted that we were asked to produce a second edition and that this provided the opportunity for updating and enhancing the original text. The justifications and rationales for writing a book about critiquing nursing research are just as applicable today as they were when we proposed the original edition. Indeed, if the number of papers published in the nursing (and health care) literature that focus on aspects of evidence-based practice are an indication, then it is evident that the rationales for writing this book are stronger than ever.

This edition retains the features which made the original a 'best seller' and we have added additional material in the hope that this expands the book's (to borrow a phrase from Tolkien's parlance) 'applicability'. In addition to reviewing and subsequently updating the material of the original text, we have added two further examples of approaches to critique along with examples. Interestingly, our extensive search identified no 'new' approach subsequent to the publication of the original text. However, these additional approaches further indicate the width and breadth of different approaches to critiquing research. Interestingly, the approach described by Polit *et al.* (2001) underpins our original arguments *vis à vis* the underdevelopment of approaches specifically designed to critique qualitative research studies, and simultaneously illustrates the work that yet remains to be done in that paradigm.

The additional chapter on how to critique research as part of the work of preparing a dissertation arose in response to the requests of students and adds further applicability to critiquing *per se*. The chapter on European psychiatric nursing research is a specific attempt to acknowledge and respond to trends in global health and international nursing, and not least, the increasing recognition that to limit one's scope to a particular country (or continent) is to set artificial and highly limiting boundaries on knowledge utilisation and knowledge transfer. Last but not least, Professor Kevin Gournay has written the Foreword to the second Edition, complementing the first provided by Professor Allison Kitson. As with the original book, we welcome feedback and comment and review and hope that such information might inform the production of a third edition.

John Cutcliffe and Martin Ward
September 2006

Reference

Polit, D. F., Beck, C. T. and Hungler, B. P. (2001) *Essentials of Nursing Research: Methods, Appraisal and Utilization*, 5th edn. Lippincott, Philadelphia.

Acknowledgements

This book could not have been produced without the sterling commitment and efforts of the Journal Club coordinators and members. Accordingly, this book is a tribute to all your hard work.

We offer thanks to Annelie Guard and the previous administrators of the NPNR for their support in maintaining the journal club.

We are most grateful to both Alison and Kevin for writing insightful endorsements in their Forewords.

To all those people who offered helpful and constructive feedback and review comment, we offer our thanks.

And not least, we offer our most profound thanks to our publisher, Helena Raeside, whose patience and industry have helped make this second edition a reality.

John Cutcliffe and Martin Ward
September 2006

Background to psychiatric/ mental health nursing research and critiquing research

CHAPTER I

The growth of evidence-based practice and the importance of critiquing research

Man's search for meaning is the primary motivation in his life and not a secondary rationalization of instinctive drives (Victor Frankl, Man's Search for Meaning, 1945)

The movement towards evidence-based practice

A son asks his father, 'How does petrol make your car work, daddy?'. The father, not wishing to confuse the little boy, and not really knowing himself, replies, 'Well, when the engine gets thirsty you put the petrol in and the engine drinks it. When it has had enough it feels better and it runs again – just like you'. The boy, not wholly convinced of this, asks further questions, so his father brings out a mechanics manual, then an encyclopaedia, and then takes the boy next door to talk to his neighbour. Finally, in exasperation, the father connects to the Internet and finds a web site that gives the answer the boy needs, at the level he needs it and in a way that not only makes sense to him but also is technically correct for his age and degree of understanding.

Many years later the boy, despite his father, becomes a mechanic. One day a customer asks him, 'How does petrol make my car work?'. If the son had learnt from his father and gone no further than making things up as he went along he would not have an answer to satisfy the customer's question. Fortunately, his studies and his training have taught him differently and he is able to provide an answer that equips the customer with the appropriate information. What is the morale of this story? Never listen to your parents? No – it is that there is an answer to every question, but sometimes you have to go to extraordinary lengths to find it and it is not possible to progress your understanding of life until you do.

How does this help us come to a conclusion about the significance of evidence-based mental health care? Perhaps more importantly, how can its implementation help individual practitioners? To answer these questions it is necessary to look back at the history of psychiatric/mental health nursing and its relationship to service development and care delivery.

As a separate speciality, psychiatric/mental health (P/MH) nursing has perhaps only a 100 year history. It was not until the 1910s that, for political reasons, those who cared for the mental ill were seen as separate from those who cared for the physically ill. The science upon which these practitioners based their actions came from a combined source: general nursing and psychiatry. As a consequence, the only thing that differentiated these practitioners from other nurses was the diagnosis of their patients. Two world wars, the increase in psychotherapeutic psychiatry, the introduction of psychotropic medications and a greater public awareness of mental illness shaped their professional actions into something akin to specialist care. However, they were under-educated, made very few clinical decisions and had little power, other than that of a subversive nature. By the late 1950s, their work was dominated by psychiatrists. Despite having their own syllabus for basic training, most of their textbooks were written for them by psychiatrists; psychiatrists sat on their examination boards; and psychiatrists dictated their working conditions and gave them clinical orders.

During this time it would have been very difficult for a mental health nurse to describe what s/he actually did. Yet do something they did, for there were in excess of 250,000 in-patient beds, and nurses were the mainstay of the daily support these people received. Over time the situation changed as nurses began to improve their own understanding of their capabilities, sought higher education, undertook research into their actions and began to share their experiences by writing about them. As they became more articulate they developed professional confidence, took responsibility for their own professional actions and began to develop a body of evidence to support their decisions. In effect, they displayed some of the traits that have been associated with being a profession (though whether or not nursing is a profession falls outside the scope of this book). They influenced the reduction of power differentials between themselves and other disciplines, contributed to general strategic and policy activities and became independent of the restricting influence of the science from which they had sprung. Crucially, nurses started to undertake and lead their own research, and thus began to develop their own unique knowledge base.

During that period of time also, mental health services matured, shedding thousands of beds, developing more therapeutic alternatives rather than relying on the myopic polemicism of community versus in-patient care, and advancing policy which would try to meet the needs of the patient rather than those of the service (Johnson and Thornicroft, 1993; Burns and Priebe, 1999). It could almost be posited that as mental health care evolved, so too did its nurses. The effects are startling. Nurses now take an active part in strategic planning, undertake a large portfolio of personal and professional research, influence clinical care and work collaboratively with service users to develop the diversity of care options necessary to meet the needs of a very specialised target population.

Evidence-based practice and evidence-based mental health care

Much of contemporary P/MH nursing practice is complicated and demands high levels of sophisticated personal and clinical technology. All of it can be complex and demanding. As described above, this shift in emphasis away from loosely defined nursing practices dictated by the actions of psychiatry to ones which form part of dedicated nursing interventions that are brought to bear as part of a collaborative multidisciplinary effort has taken place as a result of many things. One of those is the advent of evidence-based health care (Evidence-Based Medicine Working Group, 1992; Sackett *et al.*, 1996, 1997). Consequently, it is necessary to examine the key components of evidence-based practice – namely research, evidence and critiquing/critical reading of the literature – as well as locating these within the context of the development of evidence-based mental health care.

What is research?

The often quoted definition of research provided by the Department of Health (1994, p. 37) asserts that research is 'rigorous and systematic enquiry conducted on a scale and using methods commensurate with the issue to be investigated, and designed to lead to more generalised contributions to knowledge'.

Research then involves a systematic search for knowledge, and mental health care research is thus concerned with uncovering knowledge that is important (and useful) for mental health practitioners. As intimated in the Department of Health's definition, there exists a wide range of research methods and method-ologies, which are broadly grouped together under two paradigms: quantitative and qualitative. Each paradigm is concerned with uncovering new knowledge; however, the type of knowledge produced and the way the researchers go about uncovering this knowledge is different within each paradigm.

Kerlinger (1986), one of many advocates of the quantitative approach to research, asserts that the way to truth is through rigorous research, involving the identification of variables within hypotheses and subjecting them to experimental manipulation. Here 'hard evidence' is required in order to be certain that something is or is not true. To Kerlinger, this approach is at the peak of a hierarchy of how to know; further down are less respectable ways of knowing, including 'tenacity', 'authority' and '*a priori*'. The end result of each of these ways of knowing is knowledge; what differs is how the knowledge is acquired. Kerlinger has great respect for knowledge gained through the scientific quantitative method and less for knowledge gained through what he perceives as more subjective approaches. However, the importance of qualitative research, which Kerlinger would describe as 'subjective', and the different forms of evidence will be explored in more detail below.

There are commonalities between research and other related forms of enquiry, but there are important differences. Muir Gray (1997, p. 69) declares that, within the UK National Health Service Research and Development programme, these distinguishing features can be summarised as follows. Research should:

- provide new knowledge necessary for the improvement of the NHS
- produce results that are generalisable
- follow well-defined study protocols that have been peer reviewed
- have obtained formal approval from an ethical committee where appropriate
- have defined arrangements for project management
- produce findings that are open to critical examination and accessible to all who could benefit from them (and this would therefore involve publication).

Here too it is acknowledged that different approaches can be used to obtain knowledge, yet there is an intimation that quantitative approaches are favoured. Generalisation is invariably associated with randomised controlled trials, and most researchers who use a qualitative approach would not claim that their findings have nomothetic generalisability. Therefore it is possible in the above description to see plainly the influence of a quantitative way of knowing. The need to confirm and verify takes precedence within this approach. The result is hard numerical data representing reality that is then often accepted as truth and enters the knowledge base of the profession.

The historical dominance of quantitative research within mental health care

Examination of the research undertaken within the domain of psychiatry (and psychiatric nursing) indicates a historical emphasis on quantitative studies. It can be seen that from the mid-1950s onwards a large percentage of the research available to mental health practitioners centred on the trialling of medications. These drug studies were numerous but often of limited quality (Bero and Rennie, 1996; Greenhalgh, 1997a). Significantly, at first, psychiatry was only interested in quantitative studies and in particular, randomised controlled trials (RCTs). Examples of the use of RCTs in psychiatry begin to appear in the professional literature throughout the 1980s, but from the early 1990s onwards there is a marked increase in their numbers (McFarlane *et al.*, 1995; Kulpers *et al.*, 1997; Stensky *et al.*, 2000). This is because much of medical research is quantitative in nature and RCTs were regarded in the UK as the 'gold standard' of robust clinical enquiry. However, since the early 1990s those working within psychiatry and mental health care have recognised the need to use the huge amount of other forms of research and other forms of evidence at its disposal to inform its work.

Reviews of RCTs became essential during this time (Haynes *et al.*, 1996; Roth and Fonagy, 1996) because it is impractical for practitioners to read everything that has been published for themselves. Not only that, but not all the RCTs report the same results (Chalmers and Altman, 1995). Hence you might have a situation where half of a group of research projects indicate that treatment X is the best, whilst the other half suggest that treatment Y is of better value. If the practitioner only read the first group of projects s/he would be inclined to use treatment X, and likewise for those only reading papers which recommended treatment Y. Four things, therefore, occurred during the 1990s to deal with the massive increase in available research material:

- The development of models to enable individuals to appraise, in a critical manner, or review single and groups of literature papers (Greenhalgh, 1997b; NHSE, 1999).
- The development of models to undertake systematic reviews of large amounts of literature (Cullum, 1994; NHS Centre for Reviews and Dissemination, 1996; Hek *et al.*, 2000).
- The development of databases and review libraries that would make available completed reviews carried out by panels of clinical and research experts in the field (Lefebvre, 1994; Brazier and Begley, 1996).
- The development for researchers of guidelines that would inform the design and management of robust clinical trials (Medical Research Council, 2000).

In theory, these four activities should provide a framework to ensure that practitioners know how to review literature; access reviews of large amounts of literature; and have a better understanding of how to carry out and report on their work. The problem with this is that it assumes that all staff are able to access these skills, or are given them whilst they are undertaking their professional training and education, which patently is not the case. Furthermore, up until the 1990s, it was also (wrongly) assumed that the only critically sound research was that carried out using quantitative methods of enquiry for both nursing and mental health, yet this was patently not the case (Sackett *et al.*, 1997; Ward *et al.*, 1999). As Smith (1998) points out, much of mental health care is not susceptible to quantitative research methods.

The movement towards a more pluralistic approach

As a result, pressure for the inclusion of qualitative research studies and other forms of evidence to be included within the scope of evidence-based practice came from several sources, including professional academia, the social sciences, clinical psychology, nursing and medicine, particularly psychiatry. Their reasoning was obvious and contained two main arguments. Firstly, quantitative research examines known phenomena, e.g. one therapy against another, one or both of which have already been in use and are being compared to establish effectiveness against each other; or the statistical outcome value of a drug used to reduce symptoms for a recognised diagnostic entity such as one of the forms of schizophrenia. However, qualitative researchers suggest that for this research to take place the entity itself has to be placed in context, otherwise it is unclear just what the drug or therapy is acting upon. Thus, as Dodd (2001) argues, this indicates the need for preliminary exploratory, descriptive, contextual, phenomenological and anthropological studies, i.e. those which describe entities, which are the domain of qualitative research.

Secondly, and perhaps more importantly, qualitative research is not simply used to describe contexts for entities. There are known phenomena that in themselves are not susceptible to quantitative processes, e.g. belief structures, feelings and interactions (and an argument has been suggested which purports that much of psychiatric/mental health nursing may be invisible or immeasurable, and thus not accessible using quantitative methods). Thus qualitative methods are required in order to understand the nature and complexity of these phenomena. Mental health care is based upon the principles of human interactions and the ability of service users to develop personal strategies for living. True, for some there is a major role for medication and some other forms of physical therapy in this work, but essentially it is people intensive and deals with emotions, thoughts and adaptability. Similarly, as we have already described, such care is being delivered in ever-changing environments and increasingly in community settings, very often those of the patient's own home. For research to make sense of these entities and for that research to be of value to practitioners wanting to implement it in their own work it has to be environmentally and people focused. Qualitative researchers argue that these types of service, and the personal work that they undertake, are the domains of their methods.

Further evidence of embracing methodological pluralism

Even the most cursory examination of the extant methodological literature, and perhaps more significantly, the systematic review literature, will show that methodological pluralism is becoming the latest orthodoxy. Inextricably linked to this development is the growing recognition and valuing of findings from qualitative studies. Moreover, the criticisms that qualitative studies can sometimes be 'isolated' and parochial in nature is being addressed by means of a number of processes, not least the development of methods for systematic review of qualitative studies and the increasing attention given to qualitative meta-synthesis (see for example the work emerging from the various international Cochrane Centres, such as Florence *et al.* 2006; Roen *et al.*, 2006; Pluye *et al.*, 2006). At the present moment, it would be epistemologically premature to assert that developments in qualitative meta-synthesis are robust and without methodological controversy. Nevertheless, such intellectual tussles are not only useful, they are necessary. The emerging findings from these endeavours are, however, compelling and worthy of examination. Before so doing, it is necessary to remind ourselves of the nature of the generalisable findings that qualitative studies aspire to.

Qualitative researchers do not seek to generalise their findings in the same way that a quantitative researcher might. That is, they do not seek *nomothetic* generalisations relating to universal laws and absolute 'truths'. They do seek, however, to produce *idiographic* or *naturalistic* generalisations – that is, generalisations about and drawn from cases (Baskerville, 1996). Generalisations drawn from purposeful samples who have experience of the 'case' are thus applicable to similar 'cases', questions and problems, irrespective of the similarity between the demographic group (Sandelowski, 2004). In P/MH nursing studies for example, each 'case' of nursing will bear a clear resemblance to P/MH nursing as a 'whole' and any related similar 'cases'. Denzin and Lincoln (1994, p. 201) make this point most cogently when they state:

> Every instance of a case or process bears the general class of phenomena it belongs to.

Thus a process that is identified in one setting, group or population (i.e. one case), can be similarly experienced by another related setting, group or population. For example, a Grounded Theory concerned with inspiring hope that was induced from a sample of nurses is likely to be generalisable to, and bear similarity with, any population that shares the process of hope inspiration.

Work on the systematic review of qualitative studies using the Joanna Briggs Institute Qualitative Assessment and Review instrument (Florence *et al.*, 2006) perhaps illustrates the nature of idiographic generalisable findings. Individual researchers from the UK, Spain, the USA, Canada, Thailand, Hong Kong, China and Australia independently produced a meta-synthesis of qualitative studies, with 18 pairs of reviewers from diverse cultures and contexts. The results of the meta-synthesis exercise were analysed to identify the degree to which inter-reviewer agreement was achieved between these 18 pairs. In spite of the differences in background, the similarity in meaning of the synthesised findings across the participant pairs was striking. There was remarkable consistency within and between groups. Other methodological work is occurring which attempts to combine and synthesise quantitative meta-analyses and qualitative meta-syntheses (see for example, Roen *et al.*, 2006; Pluye *et al.*, 2006). Accordingly, while it remains the case that quantitative methods still hold the dominant position within psychiatric nursing research (especially if one adopts an international perspective and examines the funding/publication patterns in different countries), there are very clear signs that there is movement within the academic community towards methodological pluralism; and a parallel recognition that the psychiatric research academe needs both paradigms in order to achieve the most complete understanding possible.

What is evidence? The different forms of evidence

As indicated in previous sections, some authors regard the findings or results produced from a quantitative research study to be 'hard evidence'. Appleby *et al.* (1995) for example, intimate that evidence is reliant on the existence of (quantitative) research findings. However, as we similarly indicated in the previous section, it is important to acknowledge that a more pluralistic perspective exists. In their often quoted work, Sackett *et al.* (1996) provide a definition of evidence-based practice that does not specifically mention quantitative research. They see it as 'the conscientious, explicit and judicious use of current best evidence in making decisions about the care of individual patients'. Similarly, McKibbon and Walker (1994) offer an even less rigid definition of evidence-based practice, representing it as, 'an approach to health care that promotes the collection, interpretation and integration of valid, important and applicable patient reported, clinician observed, and research derived evidence'.

As a consequence of accepting more pluralistic views of the nature of evidence, and perhaps as a way to explain the apparent contradictions in definitions of evidence-based practice (McKenna *et al.*, 2000), hierarchies of evidence have been suggested, such as the hierarchy described in Box 1.1.

It needs to be acknowledged that such hierarchies of evidence are by no means universally accepted, particularly within mental health care. An alternative, and well accepted, view posits that research methods within quantitative and qualitative paradigms can be regarded as a 'toolkit': a collection of methods that are purposefully designed to answer specific questions and discover particular types of knowledge. To attempt to place these designs (and the evidence they produce) into some artificial and linear hierarchy only serves to confuse

Box 1.1 Hierarchy of evidence (based on Muir Gray, 1997)

- Level 1: meta-analysis of a series of randomised controlled trials
- Level 2: at least one well-designed randomised control trial
- Level 3: at least one controlled study without randomisation
- Level 4: non-experimental descriptive studies
- Level 5: reports or opinions from respected authorities

and obfuscate. If what is needed to answer a particular problem (e.g. the comparison of the therapeutic effects of two drugs) is a meta-analysis of the current studies in one particular area, then for that particular problem that is clearly the best form of evidence. Concomitantly, if what is required to answer a particular problem (e.g. what is the lived experience of experiencing violent incidents) is deep, thorough, sophisticated understanding, then for that particular problem that is clearly the best form of evidence.

Certainly there has been a gradual acceptance amongst the scientific community within health care that there is a definite role for both methodological forms (Mueser *et al.*, 1998; Fenton, 2000; Florence *et al.* 2006; Roen *et al.*, 2006; Pluye *et al.*, 2006). It is also recognised that it is necessary to undertake research that uses both quantitative as well as qualitative research and there is a growing trend for such approaches within mental health care (Gournay *et al.*, 2001; Lester, 2002; Goldney, 2002; Cutcliffe, 2005). Greenhalgh (1999) described this as the dissonance between the 'science' of objective measurement and the 'art' of clinical proficiency and judgement. She attempted to integrate these different perspectives into clinical methods, albeit for psychiatry, though the approach was certainly consistent with nursing.

In addition to the evidence produced by qualitative research studies, the definitions of Sackett *et al.* (1995) and McKibbon and Walker (1994), and Muir Gray's (1997) hierarchy, each allude to additional forms of evidence, namely reports (grey literature), opinions from experts/respected authorities, conference presentations, results from audits, continuous quality improvement initiatives and, importantly, patient-reported information. What such an extensive list clearly indicates is that the absence of formal research findings (from quantitative or qualitative studies) does not militate against evidence-based decisions. As McKenna *et al.* (2000, p. 40) state:

what is required is the best evidence available – not the best evidence possible.

Box 1.2 The systematic process of evidence-based practice (adapted from Peat, 2001)

- Define the problem.
- Reduce the problem to a series of smaller questions which can be addressed.
- Search for relevant literature, using both electronic and manual forms of literature search (including grey literature where it exists).
- Select the appropriate studies according to clear criteria.
- Critique or critically appraise each of these studies.
- Draw conclusions which help lead to clinical decisions and to implement practice.

In her systematic approach to evidence-based practice, Peat (2001) describes an eight-stage process, and an adapted version of this approach is contained in Box 1.2.

Amongst other helpful steps, Peat's (2001) approach clearly identifies the final of the three key elements of evidence-based practice: critiquing or critical reading of the literature.

Critiquing or critical reading of the literature

There appear to be a range of terms that are used to indicate the activity of reading an article, manuscript or paper in a critical manner in order to gauge the quality of the research. Throughout this book therefore, the terms *critiquing*, *critical reading* and *critical appraisal*, all of which refer to the process identified in the previous sentence, will be used interchangeably. Many authors have described this process of critiquing, for example Sackett *et al.* (1996), Sajiwandani (1996), Muir Gray (1997), Bury and Jerosch-Herold (1998), Dawes (1999) and Peat (2001). Critical appraisal should always be systematic, and according to Bury and Jerosch-Herold (1998) it is a way of considering the truthfulness of a piece of research. Peat (2001) makes similar statements suggesting that critical appraisal is the process used to evaluate the scientific merit of a study, and she argues that it has become an essential clinical tool. Critiquing a paper involves asking a series of questions of the paper in order to comment on the various components of the work. A critique then should assist the reviewer in deciding on how relevant and applicable the results/findings are (Sajiwandani,

1996). Peat (2001) goes as far as to suggest that critical appraisal skills are essential for making decisions about whether or not to change practice on the basis of the published research.

Practitioners who are inexperienced in critiquing literature occasionally make the mistake of associating critique exclusively with criticism, rather than associating critique with highlighting *both* the strengths and limitations of the work. Bury and Jerosch-Herold (1998) make this point clearly when they point out that one thing critical appraisal is not is an attempt to pull a paper to pieces. If we accept the axiom that there is no such thing as the perfect piece of research, and that this should be the starting point for the reviewer (Bury and Jerosch-Herold 1998), then the reviewer should always be able to identify a limitation of the paper. However, the important point to consider here is that there are different degrees of limitation or flaw. It is the reviewer's responsibility to decide whether or not these limitations are such that they undermine the conclusion(s) in the paper.

The second premise that should also be a starting point is that there is always something to be learned from a paper. Bearing this premise in mind should lead to a more balanced and constructive review. However, this point needs clarification. When one endeavours to produce a balanced critique, this in no way means that there should be an equal number of strengths and limitations identified. To attempt to do so would be to produce a somewhat synthetic and artificial critique. It is accepted as axiomatic that some published work is of higher quality than other work. Hence it is entirely appropriate, if not prudent, to point out each of the limitations where they exist. However – and crucially – it is equally important and appropriate to point out each of the strengths where they exist. Thus it is entirely possible, if not likely, that some reviews will have a greater emphasis on the limitations of the paper and some reviews will have a greater emphasis on its strengths.

The importance of critiquing research

It is an unrealistic and untenable position to expect that every nurse is able to, or indeed wants to, undertake research to influence practice. Much research is alien to many nurses. Understanding complex and sophisticated research methods, tools and procedures is just not something for which their training and education have prepared them. To be able to undertake good nursing research requires a secondary training as a researcher. For the vast majority of nurses such a luxury is neither required nor wanted.

However, research information and evidence drawn from other sources are increasingly influencing the path of care. Consequently, it is incumbent and necessary that all nurses recognise that they have a part to play in the development, understanding and implementation of that knowledge. Thus nurses are still expected to read scientific journals and to make sense of what they read. The little boy at the beginning of the chapter was dependent upon his father finding the information he needed to answer his question. That dependence made him vulnerable to misinformation and, ultimately, ignorant of the truth. Similarly, nurses need to be able to access the skills to find out for themselves rather than be dependent upon others for giving them the information they seek.

There exists a wide range of cogent reasons why nurses should be able to critique research literature. These reasons benefit the nurse who is undertaking the critique, the researcher or researchers who undertook the study, and the people (if any) who read the critique. Being able to critique the literature effectively:

- gives nurses the contemporary, up-to-date knowledge and evidence they need to support their decision making within the wider multidisciplinary team
- gives more nurses the opportunity to explore research and evidence-based literature to find innovative ways of expanding their own work practices
- increases the possibility of mental health nursing becoming more evidence-based and hopefully, as a consequence, providing a greater degree of best practice and care diversity for clients
- helps exchange information and facilitate debate around the research issues arising from the critique
- potentially increases the research reading audience, and as such increases the rejection of badly conducted research or poorly written papers
- allows readers to make sense of things for themselves without having to rely upon other people to do it for them, therefore giving them more independence and substantially increasing their knowledge base (because the knowledge belongs to them)
- reduces the possibility of misinterpretations being passed on by word of mouth, and so stopping good research being implemented or bad research being inappropriately used
- helps the researcher to refine the study or to develop a better study in the future
- helps another potential researcher to decide whether or not to base his/her study on the critiqued work
- helps facilitate the scientific/academic potential of a researcher towards excellence in developing his/her research skills

It has to be said that the techniques for effectively reviewing literature and research need to be learnt but they are infinitely more accessible to the novice or non-researcher than the intricacies of research. They do not teach you how to do research, but they can teach you how to make sense of it and to accept high-quality and reject low-quality research. Allowing the reader to become more discerning and to select effective literature through the process of critiquing, increases his/her enjoyment of the whole process of enquiry – a process that we have already said has been the basis for professional development in the absence of any real research skill.

The argument against the use of evidence-based practice

Evidence-based practice has its critics and commentators (see for example Freshwater and Rolfe's excellent (2005) text). Certainly, few credible practitioners would argue with the notion of producing the right care for the right condition or problem at the right time. However, this is not where the criticism lies. The difficulty rests with the nature of the evidence itself (and the debate surrounding what constitutes credible evidence), and how this evidence is used to influence practice, with mental health care in particular being one of the main areas where this causes concern.

Take the first point, that of the nature of evidence. Using the example of case management for serious mental illness, Tyrer (2000) argues that much of the research into different forms of case management has shown inconclusive results because we have been trying to identify which organisational method is best. Citing the work of Burns *et al.* (2000), Thornicroft *et al.* (1998) and Wykes *et al.* (1998), Tyrer concludes that research needs to concentrate on establishing the impact of evidence-based interventions used within service user contacts, not the number of contacts themselves. Although this is not a problem with the philosophy of evidence-based practice itself, it does highlight something of the issue surrounding what constitutes 'appropriate' evidence.

A further example of this situation exists in the use of new medications, specifically atypical antipsychotics. Geddes *et al.* (2000) for example, published the findings of a systematic review of drug trials which stated that because of their actions, atypical antipsychotics could be analysed as a single entity, in effect aggregating their scores. Despite admitting that there was poor quality of research into antipsychotic drugs, they still subjected that research to sophisticated statistical techniques and concluded, 'conventional drugs should remain the first treatment'. Prior *et al.* (2001) made an impassioned plea to clinicians to think very carefully before accepting these results and accused Geddes and his colleagues of 'bad science and worse medicine', pointing out that the six drugs reviewed had different ranges of both benefits and side effects.

The second issue, that of the use of evidence, is perhaps even more contentious for it might suggest a degree of ignorance amongst some practitioners of both research methods and the application of findings in practice. If practitioners remain relatively unskilled at critiquing research, it is possible to implement evidence that is not only poor in quality and unrepresentative of that available, but may have detrimental effects when inappropriately implemented. True, for nursing to have a genuine representative voice within the multidisciplinary team it has to be able to use evidence to support its decisions and be able to articulate that evidence to others (Barker and Walker, 2000). However, if the evidence used is of dubious quality, the nursing contribution to joint decision making is likely to be as devalued as if it used no evidence at all.

Further problems have been highlighted by McKenna *et al.* (2000). They especially draw attention to the position that evidence should *guide* practice, rather than *dictate* it. Drawing on Barbara Carper's (1978) seminal work, they make the case that at certain times nurses may draw on different types of knowledge to underpin their practice. Of the four different types of knowledge that Carper describes (empirical, ethical, aesthetic and personal), empirical knowledge refers to knowledge derived from research. Thus there may be occasions when the nurse may draw upon the other forms of knowledge despite the presence of research-based knowledge. However, as we have described earlier, such decisions can still be regarded as evidence-based decisions, given the different forms of evidence.

What is the future?

There can be little doubt that evidence-based mental health care, in whatever form it takes, will be with us in the future. The need for rational decision making, based upon appropriate evidence, has the potential to be both cost- and outcome-effective. The difficulties in implementing such a dramatic cultural change, however, must be addressed in a logical and systematic way. These difficulties are summarised in Box 1.3.

Within the existing care system there are already mechanisms and organisational procedures which both support and necessitate the use of evidence. The National Institute for Clinical Excellence (NICE), a government body established in 1999, was set up to link the clinical needs of patients with available technologies. These include drugs, therapies and interventions. The clinical effectiveness of these activities has to be founded upon evidence suggesting such impact, thus making research crucial to decisions made by the organisation. The role of NICE is to decide which innovations to use and to recommend them to UK ministers so that resources can be best managed within the health

Box 1.3 Summary of the difficulties in implementing evidence-based practice

- Ensuring that research priorities are set which produce evidence that reflects the needs of both users and organisations
- Carrying out the right research to produce the evidence required and not just easy or quick research to give inconclusive and superficial information
- Selecting the most appropriate research method/methodology for the questions being asked
- Teaching practitioners how to read and critique research and evaluate the findings
- Linking the aspirations of all mental health care disciplines to the same agenda, in effect establishing multidisciplinary research and change programmes
- Maintaining a balance between the evidence base which informs practice and the practitioners' own skill base, to ensure that they can they practice effectively when supporting empirical evidence exists, in addition to being able to perform effectively in its absence
- Recognising that research is not the only source of evidence
- Recognising and embracing the pluralistic approach to research methods/designs and the different types of knowledge they produce
- Teaching the skills of putting research into practice, i.e. rigorous and systematic practice development
- Developing networks which keep practitioners informed, on both formal and informal levels, of innovation and practice development success

service as a whole. In theory, this body should be best positioned to sift through the evidence and make decisions about appropriate change. In practice, this is difficult. The organisation has already been criticised for the way it carries out its work and to a certain degree these criticisms reflect the fundamental problems that many practitioners have with the way that evidence is used to inform clinical decision making. Smith (2001) argued that NICE is a good thing when it recommends treatments based on evidence, but not so when it denies them, despite evidence to suggest that they should be recommended. He felt that such a position was based solely upon financial constraints – that the treatment would be too expensive – in effect making a lie of evidence.

Not only must the right research be carried out to ensure that we have the most conclusive evidence, but the decisions provoked by that evidence have to be seen as reflecting the technologies available, free of bias in relation to cost and regulations, prohibiting practitioner freedom to choose the most suitable treatments. Whether or not it is possible to do this is debatable.

Conclusion

The growth and popularity of evidence-based practice over the last ten years is proof that health professionals generally strive to be as effective as possible. It does need to be acknowledged that there are problems associated with the methods used to develop the evidence base, assess its effectiveness and use it to develop practice. However, the fact remains that clinical decision making has to keep pace with innovation and we can no longer introduce ideas into practice simply on the basis that they seemed like a good idea at the time. Mental health nurses must learn to move with the times and that means availing themselves of the skills to find and make sense of the evidence available to them.

Nurses have to continue to develop their own research activities. This will provide them with a knowledge base with which to underpin their actions and give greater credibility to their decision-making processes, especially within the confines of the multidisciplinary team. The opportunities are enormous, and perhaps nursing is only constricted by its own collective imagination. Ultimately, nursing will either make a genuine contribution to the evidence base movement or simply become a passive observer of change. Individuals alone cannot affect this cultural shift. Nurses have to work together, share knowledge of both successes and failures and be prepared to take responsibility for their own actions. Networking their experiences is one significant way of achieving this, and the next chapter deals with one way of doing this.

References

Appleby, J., Walshe. K. and Ham, C. (1995) *Acting on the Evidence*. Research Paper No. 17. National Association for Health Authorities and Trusts, London.

Barker, P. J. and Walker, L. (2000) Nurse perceptions of multidisciplinary team working in acute psychiatric settings. *Journal of Psychiatric and Mental Health Nursing*, 7(6), 539–46.

Baskerville, R. (1996) Deferring generalizability: four classes of generalization in social enquiry. *Scandinavian Journal of Information Systems*, 8(2), 5–28.

Bero, L. A. and Rennie, D. (1996) Influences on the quality of published drug studies. *International Journal of Health Technology Assessment*. 12, 209–37.

Brazier, H. and Begley, C. M. (1996) Selecting a database for literature searches in nursing: MEDLINE or CINAHL? *Journal of Advanced Nursing*, 24(4), 868–75.

Burns, T., Fiander, M., Kent, A. *et al.* (2000) Effects of case-load on the process of care of patients with severe psychotic illness. Report from the UK700 trial. *British Journal of Psychiatry.* **177**, 427–33.

Burns, T. and Priebe, S. (1999) Mental health care failure in England (editorial). *British Journal of Psychiatry*, **174**, 191–2.

Bury, T. and Jerosch-Herold, C. (1998) Reading and critical appraisal of the literature. In: *Evidence-Based Healthcare: A Practical Guide for Therapists* (eds. T. Bury and M. Mead), pp. 136–61. Butterworth-Heinemann, Oxford.

Carper, B. A. (1978) Fundamental patterns of knowing in nursing. *Advances in Nursing Science*, **1**(1), 13–23.

Chalmers, I. and Altman, D. G. (eds.) (1995) *Systematic Reviews*. BMJ Publishing Group, London.

Cullum, N. (1994) Critical reviews of the literature. In: *Nursing Research: Theory and Practice* (eds. M. Hardey and A. Mulhall). Chapman & Hall, London.

Cutcliffe, J. R. (2005) Towards an understanding of suicide in First Nation Canadians. *Crisis: the Journal of Crisis Intervention and Suicide Prevention.* **26**(3), 141–5.

Dawes, M. (1999) Introduction to critical appraisal. In: *Evidence-Based Practice: A Primer for Healthcare Professionals* (eds. M. Dawes, P. Davies, A. Gray, J. Hunt, K. Seers and R. Snowbail), pp. 47–8. Churchill Livingstone, Edinburgh.

Denzin, N. and Lincoln, Y. S. (1994) Introduction: entering the field of qualitative enquiry. In: *Handbook of Qualitative Research* (eds. N. Denzin and Y. S. Lincoln). Sage, London.

Department of Health (1994) *Working in Partnership: The Report from the Mental Health Review Team.* HMSO, London.

Dodd, T. (2001) Clues about evidence for mental health care in community settings – assertive outreach. *Mental Health Practice*, **4**, 10–14.

Evidence-Based Medicine Working Group (1992) Evidence-based medicine: a new approach to teaching the practice of medicine. *Journal of the American Medical Association*, **268**, 2420–2.

Fenton, W. S. (2000) Evolving perspectives on individual psychotherapy for schizophrenia. *Schizophrenia Bulletin*, **26**, 47–72.

Florence, Z., Schulz, T. and Pearson, A. (recovered 2006) Inter-reviewer agreement: an analysis of the degree to which agreement occurs when using tools for the appraisal, extraction and meta-synthesis of qualitative research findings. *The Cochrane Collaboration*: http://www.cochrane.org/colloquia/abstracts/melbourne/O-69.htm

Freshwater, D. and Rolfe, G. (2004) *Deconstructing Evidence-Based Practice*. Routledge, London.

Geddes, J., Freemantle, N., Harrison, P. *et al.* (2000) Atypical antipsychotics in the treatment of schizophrenia: systematic overview and meta-regression analysis. *British Medical Journal*, **321**, 1371–6.

Greenhalgh, T. (1997a) How to read a paper: papers that report drug trials. *British Medical Journal*, **315**, 480–3.

Greenhalgh, T. (1997b) *How to Read a Paper*. London, BMJ Publishing Group.

Greenhalgh, T. (1999) Narrative-based medicine in an evidence-based world. *British Medical Journal*, **318**, 323–5.

Goldney, R. D. (2002) Qualitative and quantitative approaches in suicidology: commentary. *Archives of Suicide Research*, **6**(1), 69–73.

Gournay, K., Plummer, S. and Gray, R. (2001) The dream team at the Institute. *Mental Health Practice*, **4**, 15–17.

Haynes, R., McKibben, K. and Kanani, R. (1996) Systematic reviews of RCTs of the effects of patient adherence and outcomes of interventions to assist patients to follow prescriptions for medications. *Cochrane Library* (Updated 30 August 1996). BMJ Publications, London.

Hek, G., Langton, H. and Blunden, G. (2000) Systematically searching and reviewing literature. *Nurse Researcher*, **7**(3), 40–57.

Johnson, S. and Thornicroft, G. (1993) The sectorisation of psychiatric services in England and Wales. *Social Psychiatry and Psychiatric Epidemiology*, **28**, 45–7.

Kerlinger, F. N. B. (1986) *Foundations of Behavioural Research*, 3rd edn. Holt, Rinehart & Winston, New York.

Kulpers, E., Garety, P., Fowler, D. *et al.* (1997) London–East Anglia randomised controlled trial of cognitive-behavioural therapy for psychosis 1: Effects of the treatment phase. *British Journal of Psychiatry*, **171**, 319–27.

Lefebvre, C. (1994) The Cochrane Collaboration: the role of the UK Cochrane Collaboration in identifying evidence. *Health Libraries Review*, **11**(4), 235–42.

Lester, D. (2002) Qualitative versus quantitative studies in psychiatry: two examples of cooperation from suicidology. *Archives of Suicide Research*, **6**(1), 15–18.

McFarlane, R. W. Lukens, E. Link, B. *et al.* (1995) Multiple family groups and psychoeducation in the treatment of schizophrenia. *Archives of General Psychiatry*, **52**, 679–87.

McKenna, H. P., Cutcliffe, J. R. and McKenna, P. (2000) Evidence-based practice: demolishing some myths. *Nursing Standard*, **14**(16), 39–42.

McKibbon, K. A. and Walker, C. J. (1994) Beyond ACP Journal Club: how to harness Medline for therapy problems. *Annals of Internal Medicine*, **121**(1), 125–7.

Medical Research Council (2000) *A Framework for Clinical Trials of Complex Health Interventions*. Medical Research Council, London.

Mueser, K., Bond, G., Drake, R. *et al.* (1998) Models of community care for severe mental illness: a review of research on case management. *Schizophrenia Bulletin*, **24**, 37–74.

Muir Gray, J. A. (1997) *Evidence-Based Health Care*. Churchill Livingstone, Edinburgh.

NHS Centre for Reviews and Dissemination (1996) *Undertaking Systematic Reviews of Research on Effectiveness*. CRD Report No 4. Centre for Reviews and Research on Effectiveness, York.

NHSE (1999) *Critical Appraisal Skills Programme*. NHSE Anglia and Oxford.

Peat, J. (with Mellis, C., Williams, K. and Xuan, W.) (2001) *Health Science Research: A Handbook of Quantitative Methods*. Sage, London.

Pluye, P., Grad, R., Dunikowski, L. and Stephenson, R. (recovered 2006) A challenging mixed literature review experience. *12th Cochrane Colloquium*, The International Cochrane Collaboration, Ottawa. http://cochrane.mcmaster.ca/ottcolloquium.asp.

Prior, C. Clements, J. Rowett, M. *et al.* (2001) Atypical antipsychotics in the treatment of schizophrenia. *British Medical Journal*, **322**, 924.

Roen, K., Rodgers, R., Arai, L., Petticrew, M., Popay, J., Roberts, H. and Sowden, H. (recovered 2006) Narrative synthesis of qualitative and quantitative evidence: an analysis of tools and techniques. http://www.cochrane.org/colloquia/abstracts/ottawa/0-058.htm

Roth, A. and Fonagy, P. (1996) *What Works for Whom? A Critical Review of Psychotherapy Research*. Guilford Press, New York.

Sackett, D. L. Rosenberg, W. Muir-Gray, J. *et al.* (1996) Evidence-based medicine: what it is and what it isn't. *British Medical Journal*. **312**, 71–2.

Sackett, D. L. *et al.* (1997) *Evidence-Based Medicine: How to Practice and Teach EBM*. Churchill Livingstone, London.

Sajiwandani, J. (1996) Ensuring the trustworthiness of quantitative research through critique. *Nursing Times Research*, **1**(2), 135–42.

Sandelowski, M. (2004) Using qualitative research. *Qualitative Health Research*, **14**(10), 1366–86.

Smith, M. (2001) The failings of NICE. *British Medical Journal*, **322**, 489.

Smith, P. (1998) *Nursing Research: Setting New Agendas*. Arnold, London.

Stensky, T. Turkington, D. Kingdon, D. *et al.* (2000) A randomised controlled trial of cognitive-behavioural therapy for persistent symptoms of schizophrenia resistent to medication. *Archives of General Psychiatry*, **57**, 165–72.

Thornicroft, G., Wykes, T., Holloway, F. *et al.* (1998) From efficacy to effectiveness in community mental health services. PRiSM Psychosis Study 10. *British Journal of Psychiatry*, **173**, 423–7.

Tyrer, P. (2000) Are small case-loads beautiful in severe mental illness? *British Journal of Psychiatry*, **177**, 386–7.

Ward, M. F. Cutcliffe, J. and Gournay, K. (1999) *A Review of Research and Practice Development Undertaken by Nurses, Midwives and Health Visitors to Support People with Mental Health Problems.* United Kingdom Central Council for Nurses, Midwives and Health Visitors, London.

Wykes, T., Leese, M., Taylor, R. *et al.* (1998) Effects of community services on disability and symptoms. PRiSM Psychosis Study 4. *British Journal of Psychiatry*, **173**, 385–90.

CHAPTER 2

The Network for Psychiatric Nursing Research (NPNR) and the National Journal Club

Introduction

It has taken P/MH nursing about a hundred years to reach the level of professionalism that it has today (although whether or not it is a 'profession' or indeed should aspire to being one is a matter for debate; see Cutcliffe and Ward, 2006). In that time it has had to deal with social prejudice, poor resources, segregation, the absence of a substantial body of specific clinical skills which would clearly separate it from other nursing specialities, a lack of clear role definition, inter-disciplinary tribalism associated with professional hierarchies and, more recently, the recognition that sometimes it lacks evidence to support its actions. Add to that any number of organisational, legal and structural changes and it is hardly any wonder that at times its identity as an acknowledged entity has been called into question. Yet survive and flourish it has, and currently it is recognised as an essential partner in the core disciplines of psychiatric care, along with medicine and psychology. Increasingly, its responsibilities have expanded to accommodate innovation and development and it has had to accept roles that allow it to function effectively with social, as well as health, care agencies. In the UK alone there are 56,000 P/MH nurses registered with the United Kingdom Central Council for Nurses and their work activities are as diverse as the geography of the country in which they work.

However, life has changed around them and it is no coincidence that mental health care services themselves now face a series of questions about their credibility in a world that is fast becoming driven by evidence and the need to generate it. Psychiatry has been accused of lagging behind medicine generally in its attempts to establish its evidence base (Kennedy, 2000) and P/MH nursing has not fared much better (Ward, 1994; Kempster, 1998). Even where there is sufficient evidence to influence practice some authors have argued that there is not enough dissemination, and practitioners are reluctant to use it even when it is made available to them (Waddell, 2001).

Nonetheless, P/MH nursing has not achieved its success by default, nor has it relied upon the resources of psychiatry to provide it with its existing evidence base. This is all the more remarkable when one considers that, prior to 1989 and the introduction of a completely new approach to providing pre-registration nurse education (ENB, 1989), the only exposure to research and research findings that the vast majority of nurses had was through their own personal development programmes and/or the gaining of higher degrees (Hunt and Hicks, 1983). In fact, Chung and Nolan (1994) show that P/MH nurses were positively discouraged from questioning the nature and development of psychiatric knowledge up until the middle of the 1980s. Natural enquiry and the desire to get things done effectively have to a certain degree overcome these obstacles (Ward, 2000a), but despite this, in the late 20th century P/MH nursing was still attempting to make sense of what it did, and for whom (Barker, 1999; Clarke, 1999).

That period of time also saw nurses themselves question practices that had been their responsibility for as long as P/MH nursing had been available – such things as close or special observations, control and restraining techniques, the use of 'as required' (PRN) medications following untoward or violent incidents, the use of seclusion and the efficacy of counselling and/or cathartic interactions. It also experienced alarm at the way that nursing was being used to plug the gaps in acute in-patient care (Ward *et al.*, 1999) in the light of increasing shortages of suitably qualified staff (Ward, 2000b). Such self-doubt and questioning could have brought about a crisis within P/MH nursing, but it was not to be the case. As usual, individual nurses and opinion drivers rallied the others and new roles were accepted with the same enthusiasm as old ones, new organisational activities were tackled with resignation and purpose, and new responsibilities were accepted, if at times not fully appreciated. More importantly, P/MH nursing began to undertake a large portfolio of research in its attempt not only to make sense of the work that it did but also to provide the evidence to support its own actions and clinical decision making.

Development of the Network for Psychiatric Nursing Research

It was in the light of these activities that the Network for Psychiatric Nursing Research was born. Its rationale came from several quarters, but perhaps the most important was the 1994 review of P/MH nursing (Department of Health,

1994) which cited MIDIRS (Midwives' Information Resource Service) as a good example of a speciality-specific database and networking system. The review was very positive that P/MH nursing should remain a speciality rather than be subsumed into generic nursing and recommended that part of this process included the development of its own information and networking system. At the time of evidence being presented to the review body – 1993 – there was no obvious networking available for P/MH nurses and much of its research was fragmented and, at times, very personalised. Nurses tended to undertake research for higher degrees, with the result that it was often not published and consequently prone to replication. There was no way of gauging the quality of this work and even less chance of it coming together to form a substantial body of knowledge for use by the profession as a whole (Ward, 1994).

Following publication of the review a meeting was organised by one of the authors for principal UK P/MH academics and opinion leaders that took place in Oxford in May 1994. Several options were open to this group. With no previous resource available there was a blank canvas, but it was important that a network was not developed simply for the sake of it. What was needed was an organisation that would have meaning and purpose and plug a needed whole, not just any hole.

It was agreed that research had to form the basis of any new group. In the light of growing interest at that time in evidence-based practice it was seen as necessary that something was available which would promote the culture of research within P/MH nursing and offer a forum for its dissemination. It would need to be a resource for those wishing to undertake research of their own, linking those who knew how to undertake the work with those wishing to learn. It needed to offer those who wanted to benefit from the work of others the opportunity to read about, and have access to, good practice activities whilst providing a method of linking people together, and not just their work.

Though the network did not fully materialise from this meeting, certain fundamentals were agreed. The network would need to be:

- specific to P/MH nursing, though it was hoped that other disciplines involved in psychiatric care and the social sciences would use or belong to it.
- based upon research and its application to practice, i.e. practice development (these terms were used as defined in the report of the task force of the strategy for research in nursing, midwifery and health visiting (Department of Health, 1993).
- comprised of two separate components: a database holding current, intended and completed projects, plus a contact directory putting people in touch with each other for specific projects, interests, support and information.
- for submitted research work from network members and not simply a trawl of existing research published in journals or held on other databases.

- available by postal access. (At that time the cost of technology for putting the network on to the Internet was prohibitive, and email, as we know it today, was still only available to a minority.)
- organised around a specific pre-formatted menu of mental health topics enabling access to the directories.
- serviced by its own publication, a quarterly newsletter, which would be distributed to all network members.
- supported by an annual conference.
- expandable, so that in the event of new technologies becoming available or future demand changing it could remain active and relevant. Good examples of this were the necessity for Internet access and an international directory.
- used for providing live information about the state of P/MH nursing research and practice developments through a review of the work of its members. It was envisaged that much of what was submitted to the network would not otherwise be published, so such a review would provide data that was not available elsewhere.
- able to use review material to comment on mental health nursing research strategies.
- able to publish innovative work within its own publication.
- regularly evaluated to ensure that it was meeting the needs of the research and development community and responding to any changes identified.

One of the less obvious roles of the network was seen as providing a passive voice coordinating the intended work of researchers and attempting to establish some sense of focus for the body of work being undertaken. At that time it was unclear how this was to be accomplished, but later it became obvious that, while it was virtually impossible to achieve, some influence could be maintained through the newsletter and the annual conference.

Initial development

A steering group was set up drawn from those attending the initial meeting. Discussions were held with various network providers, including the Bath Information and Dissemination Service (BIDS), which provides electronic support to all UK universities, but it became clear that if the network was to follow that route it would need a substantial injection of funds. A paper was published (Ward, 1994) asking P/MH nurses to identify topics that would inform the construction of the nursing index. It had to contain terms that were both contemporary and had meaning for nurses, not just a list of items that were considered to be current. This would aid both storage and retrieval functions. Contact was also maintained with the Speciality Assurance Team of the mental health topics for the READ code project (Department of Health, 1998), who were at that time developing a similar thesaurus for the NHS, and the NHS Centre for Reviews and Dissemination.

The Network had to be fully compatible with existing and intended NHS-wide networking systems to enable free flow and exchange of both projects and material. A 57-item index was developed over a six-month period which took into consideration the medical subject heading (MeSH) used by the NHS to register projects within their burgeoning Project Registration System database (PRS). In theory this would have enabled an exchange of information between the two databases, but the reality was that the two systems were developed for different purposes (the NPNR for individual practitioners, PRS to enable large funders of research programmes to log their work) and this was never to take place. Documentation was developed around the index, and the operational mechanism designed so that the whole package would work. It was agreed that membership of the network would be via a small annual fee, both to cover individual administrative costs and to engender a sense of belonging among the members themselves. Finally the name of the network was agreed. This was not as simple a task as you might imagine. When asked, half the nurses who responded to the original call for items in the index referred to themselves as mental health nurses, and the other half as psychiatric nurses (hence the use of the term P/MH nursing throughout this book). The same split appeared on the steering committee. The term 'psychiatric' was eventually used because it was felt that this reflected more the wider aspirations of the intended network. Publicity material was constructed and funding sought.

Funding the NPNR

Funding options for the NPNR were limited by the availability of sponsors interested in P/MH nursing and who would be in a position to extend their support over a period of years. It was never going to be possible to maintain the network from membership subscriptions alone and setup costs in themselves were considerable. The network also had to be seen as independent of large companies and other professional agencies with P/MH nursing being both the focus and the beneficiary of its activities. Initial difficulties were that many potential sponsors could not see the necessity for a separate research network for P/MH nurses, and nor could some understand why nurses did not simply use existing resources or wait for those that were intended to come on stream within the next few years. There was a perception that nurses did not undertake the quantity of research that would warrant an independent network. Moreover, P/MH nurses were not seen as a priority group and indeed were not seen as making a real contribution to psychiatric or mental health research. In effect, there was a chicken and egg situation. Without a network to show the collective body of work, both completed and intended, or its application to practice, there was no clear way to identify the need to establish the network in the first place.

This situation was eventually overcome by undertaking a small review of relevant published material, relating it to the findings of the P/MH nursing review and linking both these to the developing strategies for mental health care in the UK. The key potential sponsor was the Department of Health. They initially suggested that nurses use the PRS, but as this was still being developed and the NPNR indexing system was completed and far more relevant to P/MH nursing (the intended primary user of the system) they eventually agreed to support the work. Eventually, in March 1995, the Department of Health awarded the NPNR a £50,000 pump-priming grant. This would at least enable the network to become operational and so increase the possibility of further maintenance funding in the future.

A full-time administrator was appointed, hardware purchased and database development undertaken, and the NPNR became active from July 1995 onwards.

Growth of the NPNR

One of the first tasks to be undertaken following the initial launch was to set up a system to evaluate the effectiveness and operational values of the network. In the case of the NPNR this was difficult. In the first place, its primary function was to establish a network of contacts, assemble a bank of research abstracts relating to projects and disseminate these two elements to anyone within the membership who requested them. This was achieved by virtue of the network being live and its members using it. Simply counting the numbers of members and the amount of time they used the service was deemed to be very limited evaluation because it did not tell of the effectiveness of the process. For example, if only ten people had joined the NPNR and half of them lodged a project this could be seen as a failure. However, if they kept in regular communication with each other, used each other's work to inform their own and developed a research and development programme which combined their individual talents this could be seen to be a success of the NPNR. Similarly, if the network had 20,000 members and 10,000 projects it would be seen as a major success, especially for a potential sponsor. Yet, if these members never communicated with each other or contributed to the newsletter the NPNR would effectively be failing in its primary intention – networking. To evaluate the effectiveness of the NPNR it was necessary to set up a series of secondary functions upon which its performance over time could be reviewed.

This was achieved by considering the main purpose of the dissemination process, namely:

1. The transfer and interchange of information between members.
2. The reduction of academic or research duplication.
3. The use of research to inform practice.

A series of dissemination sharing options were considered and put to the steering group for ratification, and a functional strategy was developed. Benchmarking of the NPNR was made and the first review undertaken in 2000.

The review showed that the exchange of information was the main concern of its members, with lodging projects of secondary interest. Interestingly enough, members wanted to find out about the work of others but often considered their own work to be of no value to the wider membership and were reluctant to make it available. The membership is not constant, with a core body of around 800 people changing over time and a total of nearly 2,000 who have been a member at one time or another. Three hundred projects contained within the database reflect a wide range of research interests, but to this day there are still areas of the original indexing system that have no entries. The projects themselves show that nurses have taken service developments and the organisational structures of mental health services as key areas for research, with individual interventions coming a very close second. Low on the list of priorities is research into psychiatry itself, and this is a definite shift away from what used to be the case some 15 years ago. Then nurses tended to explore areas of concern that could loosely be described as the domain of psychiatrists and possibly psychologists. It would seem that while there is still a perceived need for nurses to undertake some of this work much of their research energy has been relocated to explore the work of nurses. As such, the time when a real body of research evidence exists to support the work activities of P/MH nurses is at last becoming a reality.

The international membership has grown over the years without the necessity of introducing a separate international contact section. Seventeen countries are represented in the membership and the NPNR itself is organisationally linked to professional groups in Scandinavia, Australia, Canada and the USA. It has two web sites, one based in the UK and a Nordic group based in Norway, and most contact with the network is now via email. It publishes a quarterly newsletter, *NetLink*, which has been separately funded by sponsors and has established a base for its annual conference within Oxford University.

However, very early on in the life of the NPNR it became clear that one of the operational objectives of its work was not properly covered, either by its regular review or by the more substantial evaluation process. Dissemination is not just about the exchange of information. For it to be effective recipients have to understand the meaning of what they receive. At no time have the abstracts held by the

NPNR been subjected to a quality assurance assessment, nor is any judgement made about the quality of the research processes used to gather the data. Equally, the NPNR was never intended to replace the traditional methods of gathering information from professional journals. It was always intended that the NPNR would extend members' knowledge and/or skills rather than short-cut the system and do the work for them. A mechanism did not exist within the NPNR framework for ensuring that members were using the information they received in a constructive manner, nor was there any way of knowing whether members could independently review or critique literature. The NPNR recognised this deficiency in it workings and whilst accepting that it was not its responsibility to kite mark everything for its members, it was its responsibility to give them the skills that would enable them to make best use of the data that it contained on its databases. During late 1996 and most of 1997 work progressed on establishing a unique addition to the NPNR: a forum that would facilitate members' best use of the data, the development of its national journal club. However, before describing the NPNR's National Journal Club, it is necessary to explore the nature of journal clubs.

Journal clubs as a forum for promoting critique of research

According to Bury and Jerosch-Herold (1998), journal clubs normally involve a group of people who meet regularly to review and discuss one or several journal articles. These may or may not follow a chosen topic or theme. There is a limited literature which indicates the educational value of journal clubs. Linzer (1987) discovered that the critical skills of the members improve with journal club participation. Furthermore, Burnstein *et al.* (1996) found that journal clubs that utilise a certain structure (e.g. the use of a particular approach/model, a structured review instrument), appear to experience additional educational value. Bury and Jerosch-Herold (1998) point out that additional benefits to participating in Journal clubs include shared decision making about changes in practice; consideration of different perspectives and methods; learning from one's peers; and less sense of making judgements about work in an isolated position.

Since it needs to be acknowledged that our medical colleagues have made significant progress within the domain of evidence-based practice, it is perhaps not surprising that journal clubs are widely used by medics. Such clubs are increasingly being utilised by nurses in a variety of settings, including formal education settings. These clubs are organised using a variety of formats and need not have a fixed number of members, but do need to occur on a regular basis in order to get the maximum benefit (Morton, 1996). Clearly, clubs need an identified person (or persons) to organise the club, and sessions may derive additional benefit from having someone experienced in critiquing research take the lead in the initial meetings. The material to be critiqued needs to be distributed in advance of the club, as this allows members to read it and thus be prepared for the ensuing discussion.

The authors of this text would suggest that there is no singular correct way to run a journal club and that members will find a method that suits them best. Bury and Jerosch-Herold (1998), for example, construct the case for multidisciplinary journal clubs, whereas other clubs have been organised on a unidisciplinary basis. Selection of papers for review is clearly a decision that appears to be bound up with the composition (and discipline) of the members, and clubs should decide what, if anything, they are going to do with the 'conclusions' produced by the club.

The NPNR National Journal Club

In September 1997, the NPNR National Journal Club was launched at (uniquely for that year alone) two annual NPNR conferences held in both Oxford and Edinburgh. This journal club has several aims and purposes.

- It serves as a forum where current issues in psychiatric/mental health nursing and research can be debated, explored and discussed.
- It serves as a means of education and personal development in that each of the journal club members will have the opportunity to make a contribution. The NPNR wanted to create a forum where P/MH nurses, nursing managers, and educationalists/researchers and students could create links with one another, comment on academic developments, and have the opportunity to collate feeling and feedback about national issues in P/MH nursing.
- This would create a situation where nurses of all grades and specialities were able to exchange thoughts and feelings, network with one another (thus creating a national dialogue), review academic manuscripts and contribute to four publications a year.
- This feedback could then be used to inform national strategic developments, research initiatives and both central and local policies concerning research implementation.

How does the journal club work?

The journal club meetings are held four times a year. In order to gain a national perspective it was first necessary to involve practitioners based in each of the regional health authorities. Initially, 15 groups were established. Each of these smaller groups has an appointed Regional Coordinator (and usually some assistants) who act as a contact point for journal club members and prospective members. These individuals facilitate their regional journal club meetings, distribute manuscripts for reviews and feed back to the National Coordinator any suggestions for improvement and development.

At each meeting, all the clubs systematically review the same manuscript dealing with an issue in psychiatric/mental health nursing or research, with an opportunity for each member to contribute. Group comments are then collected at the NPNR headquarters in Oxford and condensed into a single review paper. This produces a collective national response, from both NPNR and journal club members, to the issues raised in the chosen manuscripts. This review is then published, four times a year, in the *British Journal of Mental Health Nursing* and the NPNR publication *Netlink*. Additionally, since part of the 'core business' of the journal club is critiquing research papers, all the clubs engaged in developing an approach or method that was suitable to their needs. Rather than 'wholesale' use of an existing approach, the NPNR Journal Club members wanted an approach that they felt comfortable with; that addresses the questions they want asking; and that facilitates them in their efforts to embrace evidence-based mental health care.

Choice of publications

For the first year, manuscripts were chosen by key people within the NPNR, usually in response to national issues raised by the Department of Health, UKCC, ENB, RCN or other nursing organisation. As the journal club evolved, members of the club who had a clearer sense of what the current issues were for clinicians and clients, and what changes would make the most difference to these people, made suggestions for manuscripts to be reviewed. This resulted in the choice of particular papers for review, and indeed, certain 'themes' were followed, e.g. violence and aggression. Additionally, these first 16 reviews are then used as the examples of critiques in this book. One outcome of this process of journal club members selecting the papers for review was that practitioners involved in working 'at the coal face' were able to respond (and influence) national agendas about which issues should be raised and debated.

What happens to the discussion notes produced?

Each appointed Regional Coordinator (and their assistant) collects and collates the feedback comments from the journal club meetings. These are then sent to the National Journal Club Coordinator who, together with personnel from the NPNR, sums these up in a review paper. This review, reflecting the national perspective on the issue identified, is then published in the *British Journal of Mental Health Nursing* and the NPNR publication *Netlink*. Also, if the manuscript addresses a specific issue raised by one of the national nursing organisations, then that organisation will be provided with a copy of the review. So comment will be fed back directly to the Department of Health, the UKCC, the ENB and the RCN. Comments may be also be sent on to the author(s) concerned.

Attending the journal club

All NPNR members are encouraged to attend and contribute to the journal club meetings. Additionally, members are asked to 'spread the word' and inform their colleagues of this important and exciting development. You do not have to be an NPNR member in order to attend the journal club. Currently the journal club has over 40 centres around the UK and it is hoped over the next few years that this will be extended to include feedback from international groups and members

Conclusion

The NPNR has filled a gap for P/MH nurses. It provides resources and a method of networking that were hitherto unavailable to them and it gives the opportunity for P/MH nursing research and practice developments to impact upon the delivery of mental health care. In addition it also provides a mechanism to link people together so that their work has more meaning and can be better informed, and provides them with peer support that would otherwise be absent from their personal development. Through its unique national journal club it offers a forum for discussion and debate around issues affecting P/MH nursing and its research and evolution. Journal club reviews, published in a national professional journal as well as the NPNR publication *NetLink* have the opportunity to influence the quality and increase the accessibility of the work of future writers and researchers. The NPNR continues to be the only P/MH nursing speciality network concentrating on the research activities of the profession, and there are already plans in the pipeline to increase its support of members and future members. The remainder of this book would not have been possible without the existence of the NPNR. We hope you find it useful and informative, but most of all we hope that you use it to inform your understanding of research and take your place as an active member of your P/MH nursing community.

Details about NPNR membership and events can be obtained by contacting the Network for Psychiatric Nursing Research, Royal College of Nursing Institute, Radcliffe Infirmary, Woodstock Road, Oxford OX2 6HE or visiting their web site: http://www.man.ac.uk/rcn/npnr/.

Having described the context and background to critiquing nursing research, explained the purpose and value of critiquing research, and detailed the evolution of the NPNR Journal Club, the remainder of the book is concerned with the practice of critiquing nursing research. Accordingly, the next part of the book is comprised of a range of approaches used to critique nursing research and each chapter identifies the strengths and limitations of these approaches. Each approach is also accompanied by two examples of critiques, which are based on critiques undertaken by the NPNR Journal Club (except for the reviews undertaken specifically for this second edition).

In Part 3, the book then describes the NPNR Journal Club's approach to critiquing nursing research. Since this is a developmental approach, we provide two additional examples for each of the four stages identified.

References

Barker, P. J. (1999) *The Philosophy and Practice of Psychiatric Nursing*. Churchill Livingstone, London.

Bury, T. and Jerosch-Herold, C. (1998) Reading and critical appraisal of the literature. In: *Evidence-Based Healthcare: A Practical Guide for Therapists* (eds. T. Bury and M. Mead), pp. 136–61. Butterworth-Heinemann, Oxford.

Burnstein, J. L., Hollander, J. E. and Barlas, D. (1996) Enhancing the value of the journal club: use of a structured review instrument. *American Journal of Emerging Medicine*, **14**(6), 45–50.

Chung, M. C. and Nolan, P. (1994) The influence of positivist thought on nineteenth century asylum nursing. *Journal of Advanced Nursing*, **19**, 226–32.

Clarke, L. (1999) *Challenging Ideas in Psychiatric Nursing*. Routledge, London.

Department of Health (1993) *Report of the Task Force on the Strategy for Research in Nursing, Midwifery and Health Visiting*. HMSO, London.

Department of Health (1994) *Working in Partnership: a Collaborative Approach to Care. Report of the Mental Health Nursing Review Team*. HMSO, London.

Department of Health (1998) *The Purchase of Read Codes and the Management of the NHS Centre for Coding and Classification*. HMSO, London.

ENB (1989) *Project 2000: A new Preparation for Practice*. (Pre-registration Learning Outcomes. Item 1.2.3. *The Use of Relevant Literature and Research to Inform the Practice of Nursing*). English National Board for Nursing, Midwifery and Health Visiting, London.

Hunt, M. and Hicks, J. (1983) Promoting research awareness in post-basic nursing courses. *Nursing Times Occasional Papers. Nursing Times*, **79**, 6.

Kempster, M. (1998) Evidence-based medicine in mental health. *Evidence Based Nursing*, **1**, 40.

Kennedy, P. (2000) Is psychiatry losing ground with the rest of medicine? *Advances in Psychiatric Treatment*, **6**, 16–21.

Linzer, M. (1987) The journal club and medical education: over one hundred years of unrecorded history. *Postgraduate Medicine*, **63**, 475–8.

Morton, S. A. (1996) Setting up a journal club. *Health Visitor*. **69**(11), 465–6.

Waddell, C. (2001) So much research evidence, so little dissemination and uptake: mixing the useful with the pleasing. *Evidence Based Mental Health*, **4**, 3–5.

Ward, M. F. (1994) In search of a purpose. *Nursing Times Mental Health Supplement. Nursing Times*. **90**(8), 69.

Ward, M. F. (2000a) Developing a mental health nursing network to support research. *Nurse Researcher*, **7**, 24–31.

Ward, M. F. (2000b) Campaign fails to tackle mental health staff crisis. *Nursing Times*, **96**, 15.

Ward, M. F., Gournay, K., Thornicroft, G. and Wright, S. (1999) *The 1998 Census: A Review of Acute In-patient Mental Health Services Within Inner London*. Royal College of Nursing, London.

PART 2

Examples of a range of approaches used to critique nursing research

CHAPTER 3

An introduction, and Duffy's (1985) Research Appraisal Checklist approach

Introduction

This chapter builds on the introduction to the background and context of critiquing nursing research which was outlined in Chapter 1. It is accepted as axiomatic that there is no such thing as the 'perfect' study. Consequently, one might postulate that there may, similarly, be no such thing as the 'perfect' approach to or model of critiquing research. Accepting this premise, and the need for nurses to be able to engage in critiquing research under the auspices of evidence-based practice, there are several key issues which need to be considered.

Firstly, nurses should be aware that a range of approaches to critiquing research exist. As a result, it is one of the aims of this book to introduce the reader to the variety of approaches that exist.

Secondly, accepting that there appears to be a range in the quality of the approaches to critiquing research, we have attempted to include a diverse selection and we offer our own views of the strengths and limitations of these approaches. We therefore include three well-known and three less well-known examples of such approaches.

Thirdly, nursing research has a history of being strongly influenced by the medical profession (Pearson, 1992; Cutcliffe, 1998). Thus the philosophical, epistemological and methodological beliefs of the biomedical model have been adopted by some (many) nurse researchers. As a result, positivistic philosophies, quantitative methods and the hegemony of the RCT can be seen throughout the history of nursing research. Given nursing research's historical emphasis on quantitative methods, we suggest that this emphasis can also be seen in the range of approaches for critiquing nursing research, wherein the bulk of these approaches reflect this emphasis on quantitative methods, and appear to be designed to critique the research according to certain positivistic/quantitative criteria.

Fourthly, this historical emphasis on approaches that are designed to critique a study according to quantitative criteria indicates that models of critiquing need to evolve and develop in parallel with the development of research methods and methodologies.

Fifthly, accepting the argument that approaches to critiquing need to evolve, we include a range of approaches, which when ordered chronologically familiarise the reader with the evolution of approaches to critiquing. Importantly, this issue also highlights that scope exists for additional development work in the area of approaches to critiquing, and thus this leads logically into the third part of the book, the NPNR Journal Club's approach to critiquing research.

The remainder of this chapter therefore focuses on Duffy's (1985) Research Appraisal Checklist approach to critiquing nursing research. It identifies the 51 criteria, ordered under eight major research categories, which Duffy uses as the basis for his checklist, and then provides some brief instructions on how to use the checklist when critiquing research. Following this, we provide two detailed examples (drawing on the reviews carried out by the NPNR Journal Club). Having described the approach and provided examples, we then highlight some of the advantages and disadvantages of this approach.

Duffy's (1985) Research Appraisal Checklist approach to critiquing research

Duffy (1985) suggests that in order to use his approach, the reviewer should examine each of the 51 criteria. Each of these should then be given an individual rating which best describes the degree to which the criterion is met (or not) within the research report. His rating scale ranges from 1 to 6, with 1 indicating that the criterion was not met and 6 indicating that the criterion was completely met. Duffy adds that reviewers should add brief comments to criteria that score less than 5 in order to explain the decision. Additionally, if the reviewer thinks the criterion is not applicable, then this should be marked as NA. The scores for each criterion are added together in order to give (a) a score for each separate category (e.g. a score for the abstract) and (b) a total score for the paper. Following this, the reviewer is encouraged to produce a brief summary which indicates the major strengths and limitations of the report, and this summary should reflect the scores indicated for the categories. The 51 criteria are outlined below.

1. Title			Comments
1.	The title is readily understood	123456 NA	
2.	The title is clear	123456 NA	
3.	The title is clearly related to content	123456 NA	
Category score =			
2. Abstract			
4.	The abstract states the problem, and where appropriate, hypotheses clearly and concisely	123456 NA	
5.	The methodology is identified and described briefly	123456 NA	
6.	The results are summarised	123456 NA	
7.	The findings and/or conclusions are stated	123456 NA	
Category score =			
3. Problem			
8.	The general problem of the study is introduced early in the report	123456 NA	
9.	Questions to be answered are stated precisely	123456 NA	
10.	Problem statement is clear	123456 NA	
11.	Hypotheses to be tested are stated precisely in a form that permits them to be tested	123456 NA	
12.	Limitations of the study can be identified	123456 NA	
13.	Assumptions of the study can be identified	123456 NA	
14.	Pertinent terms are/can be operationally defined	123456 NA	
15.	Significance of the problem is discussed	123456 NA	
16.	The research is justified	123456 NA	
Category score =			
4. Review of the literature			
17.	Cited literature is pertinent to the research topic	123456 NA	
18.	Cited literature provides rationale for the research	123456 NA	
19.	Studies are critically examined	123456 NA	
20.	Relationships of the problem to previous research is made clear	123456 NA	
21.	A conceptual framework/theoretical rationale is clearly stated	123456 NA	
22.	The review concludes with a brief summary of relevant literature and its implications to the research problem under study	123456 NA	
Category score =			

5. Methodology Part A: Subjects		
23.	Subject population (sampling frame) is described	123456 NA	
24.	Sampling method is described	123456 NA	
25.	Sampling method is justified (especially for non-probability sampling)	123456 NA	
26.	Sample size is sufficient to reduce Type II error	123456 NA	
27.	Possible sources of sampling error can be identified	123456 NA	
28.	Standards for the protection of subjects are discussed	123456 NA	
Category score =		
Methodology Part B: Instruments		
29.	Relevant reliability data from previous research are presented	123456 NA	
30.	Reliability data pertinent to the present study are reported	123456 NA	
31.	Relevant previous validity data from previous research are presented	123456 NA	
32.	Validity data pertinent to present study are reported	123456 NA	
33.	Methods of data collection are sufficiently described to permit judgement of their appropriateness to the present study	123456 NA	
Category score =		
Methodology Part C: Design		
34.	The design is appropriate to the study question and/or hypotheses	123456 NA	
35.	Proper controls are included where appropriate	123456 NA	
36.	Confounding/moderating variable are/can be identified	123456 NA	
37.	The description of the design is explicit enough to permit replication	123456 NA	
Category score =		
6. Data analysis		
38.	Information presented is sufficient to answer research questions	123456 NA	
39.	The statistical tests used are identified and obtained values are reported	123456 NA	
40.	Reported statistics are appropriate for hypotheses/research questions	123456 NA	

41.	Tables and figures are presented in an easy to understand, informative way	123456 NA	
Category score =			
7. Discussion			
42.	The conclusions are clearly stated	123456 NA	
43.	The conclusions are substantiated by the evidence presented	123456 NA	
44.	Methodolgical problems in the study are identified and discussed	123456 NA	
45.	Findings of the study are specifically related to the conceptual/theoretical basis of the study	123456 NA	
46.	Implications of the findings are discussed	123456 NA	
47.	The results are generalised only to the population on which the study is based	123456 NA	
48.	Recommendations are made for further research	123456 NA	
Category score =			
8. Form and style			
49.	The report is clearly written	123456 NA	
50.	The report is logically organised	123456 NA	
51.	The tone of the report displays an unbiased, impartial, scientific attitude	123456 NA	
Category score =			

Grand total =

Strengths (based on the 51 criteria) are ...

Limitations (based on the 51 criteria) are ...

> *Grand Total Score corresponding to overall categorisation of the research*
> Score between 205–306 = superior paper
> Score between 103–204 = average paper
> Score between 0–102 = below average paper

Example 1: The Network for Psychiatric Nursing Research Journal Club: Review from the 17th meeting

The paper reviewed was Parahoo, K. (1999) Research utilisation and attitudes towards research among psychiatric nurses in Northern Ireland. *Journal of Psychiatric and Mental Health Nursing*, **6**, 125–35.

Abstract/overview

This paper reports on a survey which attempted to determine psychiatric nurses' attitudes towards research, and their perceptions of their use of research and other research-related activities. The author obtained a convenience sample of 236 nurses from the six main psychiatric hospitals in Northern Ireland and from the psychiatric wards within the general hospitals. The authors states that the results of the survey show that, while the nurses report positive attitudes towards research, their perception of their use of research in practice indicates that evidence-based practice is far from being realised. The author then discusses the implications of these findings.

Note: Duffy's original maximum score is 306 (51 × 6) and consequently the overall quality of the paper is calculated according to comparison of the total score with the maximum total score. However, since Duffy includes a 'Not applicable' score for each of the criteria, it might be considered as inaccurate to consider the overall quality of the papers reviewed without taking any 'Not applicable's into account. Therefore we include two scores for each category and for each paper; one which does not take account of the 'not applicable's and one which does. We have termed this pro rata *scoring.*

1. Title		Comments
1.	123456 NA	Could have clarified what the term 'research utilization' means.
2.	123456 NA	Perhaps the title could have identified that the study was conducted only on qualified psychiatric nurses.
3.	123456 NA	Members felt that it may have been useful for the title to identify that the study was conducted only on hospital-based psychiatric nurses and not on a sample that included hospital- and community-based psychiatric nurses.
Category score = 13/18 *Pro rata* score 13/18		
2. Abstract		
4.	123456 NA	Yes – clear.
5.	123456 NA	Further details of the survey (e.g. that it used a questionnaire) may have been useful.
6.	123456 NA	The results are summarised in the main, but there appears to be some confusion regarding the nature of evidence-based practice and research-based practice (see McKenna et al., 2000), in that one can have evidence-based practice (at least in part) without the presence and application of research evidence.
7.	123456 NA	The abstract does not state any conclusions, it states only that the implications of the findings are discussed.
Category score = 16/24 *Pro rata* score 16/24		
3. Problem		
8.	123456 NA	The general problem is introduced in the second paragraph of the introduction.

9.	123456 NA	The questions are stated clearly, although the members felt they had to work through a substantial section of the paper before they reached the questions.
10.	123456 **NA**	The research question is posed as a question, not a problem statement.
11.	123456 **NA**	No hypothesis included.
12.	123456 NA	The limitations can be identified and the author makes some attempt to identify the limitations himself.
13.	123456 NA	There is an assumption in the paper that remains implicit and that is the hegemony of the Randomised Control Trial (RCT). There is a significant debate surrounding this issue (Leininger, 1992; Pearson, 1992; McKibben and Walker, 1994; McKenna *et al.*, 2000; Rolfe, 2002; Thompson and Watson, 2002). Since certain research questions can only be answered using certain research methods/paradigms (Leininger, 1992), and since different research methods/paradigms produce different types of knowledge (Dickoff and James, 1968; Carper, 1978; Benner and Wrubel, 1989; Chinn and Kramer, 1995), what is clearly indicated is that it is inaccurate to proclaim the hegemony of one method/paradigm over another. Different methods will have inherent value depending on the research question asked and the nature of the knowledge required. Furthermore, within the context of mental health nursing, the hegemony of RCTs and the evidence they produce has received additional challenge and these challenges are grounded in the notion that much of mental health nursing can be regarded as invisible and unmeasurable and thus not accessible to quantitative methods (Michael, 1994; Stevenson, 1996; Altschul, 1997; Chambers, 1998; Cutcliffe and McKenna, 2000).
14.	123456 NA	The pertinent terms are defined in part. For example, the author explores and defines the term 'research utilization', but the questionnaire that was distributed to the participants does not make such a distinction.
15.	123456 NA	
16.	123456 NA	Clearly, this is a much under-researched area and thus this study is entirely justified.

Category score = 34/54 *Pro rata* score 34/42

4. Review of the literature

17.	123456 NA	While much of the literature cited in the review appears to be either directly or indirectly related to the research question, members felt that large sections of the literature review did not appear to be particularly relevant to the study. Indeed, the extensive section of the author's paper that precedes the 'Methodology' reads much more akin to a discursive piece, exploring the relative merits/drawbacks of different methods/types of evidence for Psychiatric/Mental Health (P/MH) nurses. There is little doubt that this is an issue that warrants discussion and debate, but the members felt that much of it fell outside the context of this study.
18.	123456 NA	See comments in response to Question 17.

19.	123456 NA	Members felt that many of the studies that had been reviewed for this study had not been reviewed critically, particularly when one considers the cumulative nature of knowledge generation (Popper, 1965; McKenna, 1997), in that the author failed to show how the previous studies had subsequently built upon one another.
20.	123456 NA	The relationship of the research problem to the previous research is made clear.
21.	123456 **NA**	
22.	123456 NA	No such summary is included; however, members wondered if such a summary is warranted or indeed, common practice.

Category score = 15/30 *Pro rata* score 15/24

5. Methodology Part A: Subjects

23.	123456 NA	
24.	123456 NA	
25.	123456 NA	Members stated that they wanted more information regarding the author's remarks concerning the limited resources forcing the author into using a convenience sample.
26.	123456 **NA**	
27.	123456 **NA**	
28.	123456 NA	The subjects would be largely anonymous, however, the nursing managers would know which wards the nurses worked on and thus complete anonymity was not achieved.

Category score = 19/30 *Pro rata* score 19/24

Methodology Part B: Instruments

29.	123456 **NA**	The paper does not include reliability scores from the previous research. However, the members felt that to automatically criticise this paper on this matter would be inappropriate. Their concerns go to the use of reliability tests on surveys. Surveys, such as the instrument used in this study, are used to determine attitudes and canvas opinion, both of which can and do change over time. Given that reliability is concerned with consistency over repeated measures (Burns and Grove, 1993; Polit *et al.*, 2001; Hicks, 2004), it would be inappropriate to criticise a study on the grounds of reliability when it demonstrates that opinions have change over time. The researcher could have addressed this to some extent by repeating his survey within a short space of time of the initial survey. This may have provided the data to calculate reliability scores, but these scores would still be subject to the valid criticisms regarding opinions changing over time.
30.	123456 NA	There are no reliability scores mentioned for this current study; however, see comments in response to question number 29.
31.	123456 NA	There is no reference to the validity of the previous studies which are cited in this paper.

32.	123456 NA	The paper includes some references to validity (e.g. how content validity was achieved) and the author acknowledges the absence of current validity tests due to the paucity of previous empirical work in this area.
33.	123456 NA	

Category score = 11/30 *Pro rata* score 11/24

Methodology Part C: Design

34.	123456 NA	The design is appropriate to the study question, though scales more in keeping with measuring attitudes (Burns and Grove, 1993; Polit and Hungler, 1997; Hicks, 2004) could have been used.
35.	123456 **NA**	
36.	123456 **NA**	
37.	123456 NA	There is sufficient information to allow replication.

Category score = 10/24 *Pro rata* score 10/12

6. Data analysis

38.	123456 NA	
39.	123456 **NA**	
40.	123456 **NA**	
41.	123456 NA	Tables and figures are very clear.

Category score = 12/24 *Pro rata* score 12/12

7. Discussion

42.	123456 NA	
43.	123456 NA	This whole section of the paper was regarded by the members as strong. The members pointed out that the only limitation was the author's inclusion of results from general nurses, when he had stated that he would use only the results from the P/MH nurses.
44.	123456 NA	
45.	123456 NA	
46.	123456 NA	
47.	123456 NA	
48.	123456 NA	

Category score = 35/42 *Pro rata* score 35/42

8. Form and style

49.	123456 NA	Written in a reasonable academic style.
50.	123456 NA	The logical sequence/organisation was disrupted, according to the members, due to the paper reading akin to a combination of a discursive paper and an empirical paper.
51.	123456 NA	Tone impartial.

Category score = 13/18 *Pro rata* score 13/18

Grand total = 178

Strengths

- Clearly, this is an under-researched issue and therefore quality papers that attempt to provide such research are timely.
- The development of the questionnaire indicates an evolution of the design and methods required to investigate certain issues in this area.
- The discussion is particularly strong, and raises the relevant (and for some key) point regarding the potential reasons why P/MH nurses may not make use of research findings.
- Written in a clear, concise style and is accessible, easy to read.

Limitations

- Some of the article reads more akin to a discursive piece and the bulk of the paper reads more akin to an empirical piece of work, which perhaps causes a degree of confusion.
- The author claims to report only on the data from the P/MH nurses; however, much of the results section and discussion (to a lesser extent) reports on findings from the general nurses.
- Omits the size of the sample of P/MH nurses who were invited to participate, providing only the size of the sample who responded and the size of the overall sample (general nurses, P/MH nurses etc.).
- Perhaps contains an element of confusion between research-based and evidence-based practice.

***Grand Total Score** corresponding to overall categorisation of the research*
Score between 205–306 = superior paper
Score between 103–204 = average paper
Score between 0–102 = below average paper
Grand Total Score was 178, therefore categorised as an average paper

***Grand Total Pro Rata Score** corresponding to overall categorisation of the research*
Score between 161–240 = superior paper
Score between 81–160 = average paper
Score between 0–80 = below average paper
Grand Total Score was 178, therefore using the *pro rata* scoring method the paper would be categorised as superior.

References

Altschul, A. (1997) A personal view of psychiatric nursing. In: *The Mental Health Nurse: Views of Practice and Education* (ed. S. Tilley). Blackwell Science, London.

Benner, P. and Wrubel, J. (1989) *The Primacy of Caring: Stress and Coping in Health and Illness.* Addison-Wesley, New York.

Burns, N. and Grove, S. K. (1993) *The Practice of Nursing Research: Conduct, Critique and Utilization,* 2nd edn. WB Saunders, Philadelphia.

Carper, B. A. (1978) Fundamental patterns of knowing in nursing. *Advances in Nursing Science,* 1(1), 13–23.

Chambers, M. (1998) Interpersonal mental health nursing: research issues and challenges. *Journal of Psychiatric and Mental Health Nursing,* 5, 203–11.

Chinn, P. and Kramer, M. K. (1995) *Theory and Nursing: A Systematic Approach.* CV Mosby, St Louis.

Cutcliffe, J. R. and McKenna, H. P. (2000) Generic nurses: the nemesis of psychiatric/mental health nursing? *Mental Health Practice,* 3(9), 10–14.

Dickoff, J. and James, P. (1968) A theory of theories: a position paper. *Nursing Research,* 17, 3.

Hicks, C. (2004) *Research Methods for Clinical Therapists: Applied Project Design and Analysis.* Churchill Livingstone, Edinburgh.

Leininger, M. (1992) Current issues, problems and trends to advance qualitative paradigmatic research methods for the future. *Qualitative Health Research,* 2(4), 392–415.

McKenna, H. P. (1997) *Nursing Theory and Models.* Routledge, London.

McKenna, H. P., Cutcliffe, J. R. and McKenna, P. (2000) Evidence based practice: demolishing some myths. *Nursing Standard,* 14(16), 39–42.

McKibbon, K. A. and Walker, C. J. (1994) Beyond ACP journal club: How to harness Medline for therapy problems. *Annals of Internal Medicine,* 121(1), 125–7.

Michael, S. (1994) Invisible skills. *Journal of Psychiatric and Mental Health Nursing,* 1, 56–7.

Pearson, A. (1992) Knowing nursing. In *Knowledge for Nursing Practice* (eds. K. Robinson and B. Vaughan), pp. 213–26. Butterworth-Heinemann, Oxford.

Polit, D. F. and Hungler, B. P. (1997) *Essentials of Nursing: Methods, Appraisal and Utilisation,* 4th edn. Lippincott, Philadelphia.

Polit, D. F., Beck, C. T. and Hungler, B. P. (2001) *Essentials of Nursing Research: Methods, Appraisal and Utilization,* 5th edn. Lippincott, Philadelphia.

Popper, K. (1965) *Conjectures and Refutations: the Growth of Scientific Knowledge.* Harper & Row, New York.

Rolfe, G. (2002) A response to Thompson and Watson. *Nurse Education Today,* 22, 275–7.

Stevenson, C. (1996) Taking the pith out of reality: a reflexive approach for psychiatric nursing research. *Journal of Psychiatric and Mental Health Nursing,* 3, 103–10.

Thompson, D. and Watson, R. (2002) A response to Gary Rolfe. *Nurse Education Today,* 22, 273–4.

Example 2: The Network for Psychiatric Nursing Research Journal Club: Review from the 14th meeting

The paper reviewed was Pullen, L., Modrcin-Talbot, M. A., West, W. R. and Meunchen, R. (1999) Spiritual high versus high on spirits: Is religiosity related to adolescent drug abuse? *Journal of Psychiatric and Mental Health Nursing,* 6, 3–8.

Abstract/overview

This paper attempted to investigate the relationship between alcohol/drug abuse and the frequency of religious service attendance in adolescents within the south-eastern USA. The authors collected data, using a survey, from a total sample of 217 adolescents (aged 12–19). This sample was comprised of both a non-clinical and a clinical group. Their results indicate that as attendance at religious services increased, alcohol and drug abuse decreased. They conclude that spirituality is a concept that warrants further study in order to determine if its inclusion within treatment programs could help enhance recovery or reduce recidivism.

Note: Duffy's original maximum score is 306 (51 × 6) and consequently the overall quality of the paper is calculated according to comparison of the total score with the maximum total score. However, since Duffy includes a 'Not applicable' score for each of the criteria, it might be considered as inaccurate to consider the overall quality of the papers reviewed without taking any 'Not applicable's into account. Therefore we include two scores for each category and for each paper; one which does not take account of the 'not applicable's and one which does. We have termed this pro rata *scoring.*

1. Title		Comments
1.	123456 NA	The members felt the title was easily understood, although some wondered what the authors meant by the term 'religiosity'.
2.	123456 NA	The members felt the title was clear.
3.	123456 NA	
Category score = 15/18 *Pro rata* score 15/18		
2. Abstract		
4.	123456 NA	It was noted that, within the abstract, the relationship is stated, however, there is no reference to a research problem. Members felt that the abstract was clear and concise. Indeed, some expressed the view that the authors could have included more relevant detail within the abstract without it becoming too long.
5.	123456 NA	The abstract states that a survey was used, but perhaps it could also have provided some information on the type of survey; while it does indicate that the data was analysed, it doesn't indicate how.
6.	123456 NA	The results are summarised, albeit, very briefly.
7.	123456 NA	Members pointed out that the abstract could have contained more detail about the findings, the discussion and the conclusions.
Category score = 20/24 *Pro rata* score 20/24		
3. Problem		
8.	123456 NA	

9.	123456 NA	The questions are stated clearly, although the members felt they had to work through a substantial section of the paper before they reached the questions.
10.	123456 **NA**	The research question is posed as a question, not a problem statement.
11.	123456 NA	The hypotheses are included at the start of the 'Methods' section and are stated clearly. However, some members did wonder if the 'Methods' section was the most appropriate place for the research hypotheses.
12.	123456 NA	There did not appear to be a section that referred to the limitations of the study, and that in itself was regarded as a significant limitation of this study by the members.
13.	123456 NA	There is an assumption in the paper that remains implicit, and that is the authors' apparent belief that attendance and/or participation at religious activities (e.g. church attendance) is inherently a 'healthy' activity. Members noted that all of the literature cited in the review indicated 'positive' outcomes. Additionally, the authors draw upon certain grand theories (e.g. Roy's Adaptation model, 1980) in order to illustrate the value of engaging in 'religious' activity. Consequently, members wondered if such a selection of literature provided a balanced and objective view of the substantive area, and felt that it indicted the possible presence of the authors' assumptions. Now while there is an abundance of literature that lends support to the argument of attending to one's 'spiritual' needs (Dyson et al 1997, Walter 1997, Brandon 1999) and there is evidence that such needs can be met by engaging in 'religious' activities, it would be inaccurate to consider religious activities as the *only* way of meeting such needs.
14.	123456 NA	
15.	123456 NA	Members noted that while the author draws attention to the body of literature regarding the inappropriate use of drugs/alcohol, it was felt that a summary of the key problems such behaviours provoke would have been useful.
16.	123456 NA	Within the literature review, the authors include a comprehensive précis of the research within this substantive area. Indeed, the current extent of understanding revealed in this literature appears to indicate that the relationship between drug/alcohol abuse and 'religiosity' is very well established. Consequently, members were left wondering why it was necessary to undertake another study to further confirm that which already appears to be known, particularly when many unanswered yet relevant questions within this substantive area remain. For example, why and how does increased 'religiosity' make a difference in drug/alcohol abuse? What intra- and inter-personal dynamics occur (if any!) within this complex process that helps prevent drug/alcohol abuse?
	**Category score = 29/54 *Pro rata* score 29/48**	
	**4. Review of the literature**	
17.	123456 NA	

18.	123456 NA	Members pointed out that the literature included in the review indicated that the relationship between drug/alcohol abuse and religiosity was already well established and well researched. Consequently, the literature did not appear to indicate a need for this research question, but perhaps was a strong indication of the need for other relevant questions.
19.	123456 NA	Members felt that many of the studies that had been reviewed for this study had not been reviewed critically, but had been reported.
20.	123456 NA	This was a difficult area to assess. The relationship of the research problem to the previous research is clear, in that this study appears to be very similar to the studies that have already been undertaken. However, how this study builds upon these earlier studies (and this is another aspect of the relationship between previous and current empirical work – see Popper, 1965; McKenna, 1997) is not made clear.
21.	123456 NA	
22.	123456 NA	No such summary is included; however, members wondered if such a summary is warranted or indeed, common practice.

Category score = 19/30 Pro rata score 19/24

5. Methodology Part A: Subjects

23.	123456 NA	
24.	123456 NA	The authors do not appear to justify any of their choices in their sampling frame and this might have enhanced the paper (Morse, 1991; Streubert and Carpenter, 1999). For example, members wondered, was this a convenience sample? Why the differences in sample size for each group? Did all the non-clinical subjects attend the same church?
25.	123456 NA	Members stated that they felt the authors could have indicated more clearly their particular reasons for the sampling choices they made.
26.	123456 **NA**	
27.	123456 **NA**	
28.	123456 NA	It was noted that formal ethical approval was granted, and this is to the betterment of the paper. However, the paper contained no indication of the ethical issues or considerations, and such an inclusion might have enhanced the quality of the paper (Schrock, 1991; Burnard and Chapman, 2003).

Category score = 11/36 Pro rata score 11/24

Methodology Part B: Instruments

29.	123456 NA	
30.	123456 NA	Members pointed out that the paper did not appear to contain any information regarding reliability or validity of this study, or previous studies. As a result this was regarded as a significant limitation.
31.	123456 NA	
32.	123456 NA	
33.	123456 NA	

Category score = 5/30 Pro rata score 5/30

Methodology Part C: Design		
34.	123456 NA	The design was appropriate to the study question and provided some data that would enable the hypotheses to be tested. However, given the wide range of confounding variables and interactions of variables that could impact on patterns of drug/alcohol use, and the relationship with religiosity, it is debatable that the method used provided the clearest and most meaningful results. For example, there are arguments that posit drug/alcohol use as a symptom of a disease (i.e. addiction as a disease, Gerace 1988), arguments that indicate the social, economic, political and cultural factors as the basis for explaining drug/alcohol abuse (see Williams and Harris-Reid, 1999) and arguments for/against harm reduction rather than abstinence models (Duff, 2003; Ksobiech, 2003; Lewis, 2004). Given the possible interaction of these and other influences on drug/alcohol abuse, the members doubted that the design used in this study provided the clearest and most meaningful results. Therefore, as an alternative, the researchers might have might have considered a qualitative method. The choice of a qualitative method would have enabled the researchers to ask the clients: 'Tell me about your experiences of/attitudes towards drug/alcohol use and how religiosity effects these?'.
35.	123456 **NA**	
36.	123456 **NA**	
37.	123456 NA	
Category score = 10/24 *Pro rata* **score 10/12**		
6. Data analysis		
38.	123456 NA	This whole section was felt to be very clear, relevant and appropriate, and was regarded as a strength of the paper.
39.	123456 NA	
40.	123456 NA	
41.	123456 NA	
Category score = 24/24 *Pro rata* **score 24/24**		
7. Discussion		
42.	123456 NA	
43.	123456 NA	Members felt that, on first consideration, it appears as though the conclusions are substantiated by the evidence presented. However, as indicated previously, it was also regarded as somewhat simplistic to posit a direct inverse correlation between an increase in religiosity with a corresponding decrease in drug/alcohol abuse. Since the authors appeared to have made no attempt to isolate the dependent variable and control other influencing variables, the change in drug/alcohol use may be attributed to increased religiosity; but it may be attributed to any number of confounding variables (or a combination of these variables) (see Burns and Grove, 1993; Polit and Hungler, 1997; Hicks, 2004). Consequently, while it would be appropriate to suggest the presence of a correlation, it might have been prudent for the authors not to make such an assertive claim, particularly given the limitations of the study.

44.	123456 NA	There did not appear to be any discussion of the methodological problems.
45.	123456 NA	
46.	123456 NA	Members stated that the paper did discuss the implications of the findings to a degree. However, this discussion was limited and furthermore perhaps provided further evidence of the authors' implicit assumption/belief that attendance and/or participation at religious activities (e.g. church attendance) is inherently a 'healthy' activity.
47.	123456 NA	
48.	123456 NA	The authors do indicate the need for some additional research, but members felt there were additional questions and issues that warrant investigation which do not appear to be indicated in this paper. For example, what is it about the process and interaction of engaging in religiosity that makes a difference to drug/alcohol use?

Category score = 29/42 *Pro rata* score 29/42

8. Form and style

49.	123456 NA	Written in a reasonable academic style.
50.	123456 NA	
51.	123456 NA	Members felt that the tone of the paper was rather biased towards the view/belief that attendance and/or participation at religious activities (e.g. church attendance) is inherently a 'healthy' activity, and therefore should be encouraged.

Category score = 12/18 *Pro rata* score 12/18

Grand Total = 174

Strengths

- Many of the terms used within the paper are clearly defined.
- The paper is succinct and contains no unnecessary text.
- The data analysis section was regarded as being particularly strong.
- Written in a clear, concise style and is accessible, easy to read.

Limitations

- The paper did not appear to contain a section that referred to the limitations of the study.
- The study appeared to be very similar to previous empirical work undertaken in this substantive area, and consequently questions were asked regarding 'Does this study contribute anything new or "fresh" to the knowledge base?'.
- The omission of reliability and validity scores was regarded as a significant limitation.
- The study appears to posit a rather simplistic, linear relationship between alcohol/drug abuse and religiosity, and there is a large body of evidence that suggests

drug/alcohol use or abuse are very complex, multidimensional problems.
- The paper appeared to contained an implicit bias or assumption that attendance to, or participation in religious activities is a 'healthy' activity.

Grand Total Score corresponding to overall categorisation of the research
Score between 205–306 = superior paper
Score between 103–204 = average paper
Score between 0–102 = below average paper
Grand Total Score was 174, therefore categorised as an average paper

---

Grand Total* Pro Rata *Score corresponding to overall categorisation of the research
Score between 177–264 = superior paper
Score between 89–176 = average paper
Score between 0–88 = below average paper
Grand Total Score was 174, therefore using the *pro rata* scoring method, the paper would be categorised as average (almost superior).

References

Brandon, D. (1999) Mental health and spirituality: two survivors. *Mental Health Practice*, **2**(6), 16–19.

Burnard, P. and Chapman, C. (2003) *Professional and Ethical Issues in Nursing*, 3rd edn. Baillière Tindall, London.

Burns, N. and Grove, S. K. (1993) *The Practice of Nursing Research: Conduct, Critique and Utilization*, 2nd edn. WB Saunders, Philadelphia.

Duff, C. (2003) The importance of culture and context: rethinking risk and risk management in young drug using populations. *Health, Risk and Society*, **5**(3), 285–99.

Duffy, M. (1985) A research appraisal checklist for evaluating nursing research reports. *Nursing and Healthcare*, **6**(10), 539–47.

Dyson, J., Cobb, M. and Forman, D. (1997) The meaning of spirituality: a literature review. *Journal of Advanced Nursing*, **26**, 1183–8.

Gerace, L. M. (1993) Addictive behaviour. In: *Mental Health – Psychiatric Nursing: a Holistic Life-Cycle Approach*, 3rd edn (eds. R. P. Rawlins, S. R. Williams, and C. K. Beck), pp. 357–81. Mosby, St Louis.

Hicks, C. (2004) *Research Methods for Clinical Therapists: Applied Project Design and Analysis*. Churchill Livingstone, Edinburgh.

Ksobiech, K. (2003) A meta-analysis of needle sharing, lending and borrowing behaviours of needle exchange program attenders. *AIDS Education and Prevention*, **15**(3), 257–68.

Lewis, L. M. (2004) Culturally appropriate substance abuse treatment for parenting African American women. *Issues in Mental Health Nursing*, **25**, 451–72.

McKenna, H. P. (1997) *Nursing Theory and Models*. Routledge, London.

Morse, J. M. (1991) Strategies for sampling. In: *Qualitative Nursing Research: a Contemporary Dialogue* (ed. J. M. Morse), pp. 127–45. Sage, London.

Polit, D. F. and Hungler, B. P. (1993) *Essentials of Nursing Research: Methods, Appraisal and Utilization*, 3rd edn. Lippincott, Philadelphia.

Popper, K. (1965) *Conjectures and Refutations: the Growth of Scientific Knowledge*. Harper & Row, New York.

Roy, C. (1980) The Roy adaptation model. In: *Conceptual Models for Nursing Practice*, 2nd edn (eds. J. P. Riehl and C. Roy), pp. 179–89. Appleton-Century-Crofts, New York.

Schrock, R. (1991) Moral issues in nursing research. In: *The Research Process in Nursing*, 2nd edn (ed. D. F. S. Cormack), pp. 30–9. Blackwell Science, London.

Streubert, H. J. and Carpenter, D. R. (1999) *Qualitative Research in Nursing: Advancing the Humanistic Imperative*, Lippincott, London.

Walter, T. (1997) The ideology and organisation of spiritual care: three approaches. *Palliative Medicine*, **11**, 21–30.

Williams, D. R. and Harris-Reid, M. (1999) Race and mental health: emerging patterns and promising approaches. In: *A Handbook for the Study of Mental Health: Social Contexts, Theories and Systems* (eds. A. V. Horwitz and T. L. Scheid), pp. 295–314. Cambridge University Press, Cambridge.

Critique and summary: strengths and limitations of Duffy's (1985) Research Appraisal Checklist approach to critiquing nursing research

Strengths

- The approach follows a logical sequence, one which often mirrors that of the paper reviewed (particularly if the paper uses a quantitative method), and this makes it straightforward to follow.

- The approach produces a numerical value, which Duffy argues is representative of the overall quality of the paper, and this 'numerical' approach may be favoured by some; e.g. for many years educationalists within nursing have ascribed a numerical value to provide an indication of the quality of work.

- It is possible that the author of the research paper reviewed may learn from a critique using Duffy's approach, particularly if the reviewers include extensive comments rather than focusing on the score.

- The approach does enable both the strengths and the limitations of a study to be identified.

- The approach allows room for data and/or argument to be introduced to support the reviewer's criticisms/observations and suggestions for improvement. However, again this relies on the reviewer making extensive use of the 'Comments' section and not relying on the 'score'.
- The approach does lead the reviewer towards considering the implications of the study, but perhaps greater emphasis could have been placed on this.

Limitations

- Tends to ascribe high scores and thus indicate that papers are of high quality, whereas the views of the members of the papers would not indicate such a result.
- Clearly orientated towards evaluating quantitative studies and thus may not be appropriate (or have only limited application) for evaluating qualitative studies.
- The approach ascribes an equal weighting to each of the criteria and this may not be appropriate. For example, there may be certain criteria that are more important than others.
- The lack of guidance on whether or not the total score should or should not include the items regarded as 'Not applicable' is rather confusing.
- There are significant problems with (and a concomitant debate surrounding) the practice of assigning a numerical value to a judgement of quality. While it has to be acknowledged that educationalists have been doing exactly that for many years when they ascribe a numerical value to a student's assignment, the process is still problematic. For example, the approach has an unequal distribution of Duffy's 51 separate criteria within his categories. The section on 'Analysis' contains four criteria, whereas the sections on 'Method' contain a total of 15 criteria. This raises questions such as whether Duffy implies that the 'Method' section is nearly four times as valuable than the 'Analysis' to the overall quality of the study.
- Further problems with the scoring system include: where bands of scoring exist (e.g. 204 = average research and 205 = superior research) the addition or subtraction of one or two points can make the difference between superior and average research. Such simplistic margins suggest that explicit demarcations exist between average and superior research, and the authors of this book would argue that this is not the case. The approach does not indicate how the scores and demarcations were derived.
- The approach might be regarded as a form of simplistic reductionism, wherein a crude attempt is made to reduce the research to its simplest constituent parts, and then the reviewer attempts to 'measure' these parts.

References

Cutcliffe, J. R. (1998) Is psychiatric nursing research barking up the wrong tree? *Nurse Education Today*, **18**, 257–8.

Pearson, A. (1992) Knowing nursing. In *Knowledge for Nursing Practice* (eds. K. Robinson and B. Vaughan), pp. 213–26. Butterworth-Heinemann, Oxford.

Duffy, M. (1985) A research appraisal checklist for evaluating nursing research reports. *Nursing and Healthcare*, **6**(10), 539–47.

CHAPTER 4

Burns and Grove's (1987) critical appraisal approach to critiquing nursing research

This chapter focuses on Burns and Grove's (1987) approach to critiquing nursing research. Burns and Grove posit that there are different academic 'levels' of research critiquing which correspond to the academic levels of the nurse qualification. Accordingly, each of these different levels of critiquing involves different processes. However, the guidelines are applicable whatever level of critiquing the reviewer is aiming for. Therefore this chapter outlines their guidelines for conducting a research critique and then paraphrases the key questions the reviewer should ask, under key headings/areas identified by Burns and Grove. Following this we provide two detailed examples (drawing on the reviews carried out by the NPNR Journal Club). Having described the approach and provided examples, we then highlight some of the advantages and disadvantages of this approach.

Burns and Grove argue that there are eight guidelines which a reviewer should remain mindful of when conducting a critique, and they describe these as:

1. Read and critique the entire study.
2. Examine the research and clinical expertise of the authors.
3. Examine the organisation and presentation of the research report.
4. Identify strengths and weaknesses.
5. Provide specific examples of strengths and weaknesses.
6. Be objective and realistic in identifying the study's strengths and weaknesses.
7. Suggest modifications for future studies.
8. Evaluate the study.

Burns and Grove also identify five different levels of critiquing research, and they link these with specific levels of academic qualification:

1. Comprehension
2. Comparison
} Baccalaureate level

3. Analysis   Masters level

4. Evaluation
5. Conceptual clustering
} Doctorate/experienced researcher

Note: It is interesting to note that within Burns and Grove's description of the levels of critiquing research/academic level of qualification, there is no reference to Diploma level studies. This may be a reflection of the different patterns of nurse education between Britain and the USA. However, if we accept Burns and Grove's description then the implicit implication is that the large majority of nurses within Britain would not need any comprehension of or skills in critiquing nursing research, since the large majority of nurses in Britain have either undertaken a Diploma- or certificate-level pre-registration qualification. Clearly, this is at odds with the emphasis on evidence-based practice (see Chapter 1). Therefore we argue that it is incumbent on all practising nurses to have some understanding of approaches to critiquing nursing research, irrespective of the level of their academic preparation.

Paraphrased questions the reviewer should ask, under key headings/areas identified by Burns and Grove

1. Research problems and hypothesis
   A Is the problem clearly stated?
   B Are the key variables identified?
   C Are the hypotheses clearly stated?
2. Review of the literature
   A Were investigators suitably qualified?
   B Are classic/other studies cited?
   C Is the review logical and organised?
   D Has related literature being explored?
3. Variables
   A What variables are defined?
   B Are there any undefined variables?
   C Are independent and dependent variables clearly delineated?
4. Research design
   A Is the design clearly indicated?
   B Is it appropriate?

    C How does the design control threats to validity?

    D Could others replicate the study?

5. Research instruments

    A Are data-collecting instruments clearly defined?

    B Are the instruments appropriate?

    C Are they valid and reliable?

    D Are limitations addressed?

6. Measurement

    A Is the level of measurement described?

    B Are there data to support reliability and validity measures?

7. Sampling

    A Is the sampling procedure clearly described?

    B Is the sample random or non-random?

    C Is the sample size adequate?

8. Analysis of data

    A Are statistical values reported?

    B Was the most effective statistic chosen?

    C Was the level of significance reported?

9. Interpretation of results

    A Are the results grounded in the data?

    B Are weaknesses in the data honestly addressed?

    C Are conclusions justified?

10. Report of the results

    A Does the title of the study reflect the key variable?

    B Is there a clear abstract?

    C Has the investigator been honest?

    D Is non-sexist language used?

    E Is the report interesting?

11. Protection of human rights

    A Are procedures ethical?

    B Is informed consent obtained?

    C Are privacy and anonymity safeguarded?

Example 3: The Network for Psychiatric Nursing Research Journal Club: Review No. 13

The paper reviewed was Hannigan, B. (1999) Education for community psychiatric nurses: content, structure and trends in recruitment. *Journal of Psychiatric and Mental Health Nursing*, **6**, 137–45.

Abstract/overview

This paper reported on a survey which was designed to measure aspects of Community Psychiatric Nursing (CPN) education in the UK. It indicates that 32 of the 39 course leaders who ran post-qualifying programmes for CPNs responded to a nine-page postal questionnaire. Findings indicated that the majority of courses are now run at degree level; most courses appeared to include education in key areas of specialist content pertinent to contemporary CPN practice (e.g. collaborative working with service users). Overall, however, the paper reported that courses for CPNs appeared to be characterised by considerable variation in specialist content. The paper concludes by offering possible explanations for this variation and some suggestions for future research.

IA Within the 'Introduction' of the paper, the author describes the primary aim of the study, which was to investigate the specialist content of CPN courses currently available in the UK. However, the aim of the study is not phrased as a 'problem'. Members wondered if this was because the focus of the research was not an actual problem. Consequently, questions were raised concerning whether or not the study was required, particularly given that a similar study (with similar aims) had been carried out each year for most of the previous ten years. Alternative views were raised which indicated the value in monitoring the trends in nurse education, including CPN education, since educational curricula should, at least in part, reflect the needs of the local population and current national policies and agendas (Parkes, 1997; Norman, 1998).

IB As the study uses a survey design, and thus was not concerned with measuring causal relationships between variables, no key variables are mentioned in the study, and this was regarded as appropriate by the members.

IC The paper did not posit a hypothesis or a null hypothesis. Again, given that the research used a straightforward survey design, it was appropriate for the researcher not to include a hypothesis (Polit and Hungler, 1997; Hicks, 2004.)

2A The reported piece of research was carried out as the dissertation for a Master's degree. Given that the author had a Bachelor's degree, and had access to supervision from senior researchers, and that the research used a straightforward survey design and minimal amount of statistics in the analysis, members felt that the investigator was suitably qualified to undertake the study.

2B The study appropriately describes, and subsequently draws upon, the previous studies carried out to determine the extent of, and trends in, CPN education.

2C Members stated that the literature review was well organised and logical.

2D In addition to drawing on the literature mentioned in 2B, the author also includes some of the discursive texts which consider positions and arguments regarding the developments in CPN education. However, members wondered if the author had considered drawing upon a slightly wider literature, which might have been relevant to this issue. For example, White and Brooker's (1998) CPN surveys; literature that has examined alternative developments in CPN education, e.g. 'Thorn' training (Gamble, 1995); or the crucial role of Clinical Supervision within Community Nurse practice and education (Kelly *et al.*, 2001).

3A/B/C As this study used a straightforward survey design, and thus was not attempting to test or measure the relationship between variables, no variables were highlighted.

4A The author stated that he used a postal questionnaire which was distributed to each education centre that provided CPN courses. Therefore members felt that the design was clearly stated.

4B In order to obtain information, which can be expressed in numerical form from a wide population, a survey design is appropriate (Parahoo, 1997). Consequently, the members felt that the design used by the author was appropriate.

4C The paper does not make any reference to threats to validity. However, members constructed an argument that indicated that to automatically criticise this paper on this matter might be inappropriate. Their concerns go to the use of reliability tests on surveys. Surveys, such as the instrument used in this study, used to determine 'concrete' matters that are not 'open to debate' (e.g. the number of nurses on a course, whether or not the nurses are studying for a degree or a diploma), but which also aim to compare the changes of these figures over time, may not be best considered in terms of reliability. Given that reliability is concerned with consistency over repeated measures (Behi and Nolan, 1995; Stuppy, 1998; Hicks, 2004), it might be inappropriate to criticise a study on the grounds of reliability when it demonstrates that numbers of nurses on courses fluctuates from year to year.

Where surveys are attempting to measure less 'concrete' variables or phenomena, then it may be prudent for authors to address this by repeating the survey within a short space of time of the initial survey. This would then provide the data to calculate reliability scores. However, members felt that there were no such fluctuating variables within this paper.

4D Given the precise nature of the detail included in this paper (e.g. sample composition, design), and the fact that this study is, in the main, a replication of a study that has been conducted almost every year for the last ten years, members stated that it would be relatively easy and entirely plausible for others to replicate the study.

5A/B Members stated that the description of the survey gave them a clear indication of the nature and type of questions asked. However, the question was raised why the instrument did not include any questions about the clinical component of the courses. Since these courses appear to have been designed purposefully, blending theoretical and clinical input, one could argue that the nature of the clinical input to CPN education and training is relevant and important. Consequently, any study that intends to gain a more complete understanding of the content, structure and trends in CPN education may benefit from investigating the clinical input in addition to the theoretical input.

5C The paper does not make any reference to the validity of the instrument. Again, given that the instrument was based on one that was used in previous studies, members felt that the author could have used data from the previous studies to indicate/ determine the validity. Furthermore, the additional work carried out to extend the instrument may have benefited from some consideration of content or face validity (Polit and Hungler, 1997).

5D The author did make reference to the limitations regarding the absence of any questions in the survey pertaining to the clinical input on a course.

6A The report states that 'measurements' used in the survey were 'self reported' measures, for example self reports of the number of hours in the course, self reports on the number of the students.

6B The arguments regarding validity and reliability have been made earlier in this chapter.

7A Members stated that the sampling strategy could be regarded as one of the strengths of the paper since it sampled the total population (i.e. each education centre that provided the CPN course.) Furthermore, it achieved a response rate of 82%, which is high for a postal return survey; therefore, the members felt that such results could be taken to be indicative or representative of the total population.

7B The sample was not random, but since the study sampled the entire population, a randomised sample was not required.

7C As stated above, the sample size was considered to be highly adequate.

8A The paper utilised statistics in only a very limited way, in that percentages were used. Members felt that this was appropriate given the design of the study, and the inclusion of any unnecessary statistics might indicate an attempt to gain 'pseudo-scientific credibility' for the paper without adding anything of real substance.

8B/C There were no statistical tests carried out and correspondingly, no mention of levels of significance.

9A/B Members felt that this section could be regarded as another strength of the paper as the author appears to 'ground' his results in the data and does not appear to have 'conjured' or manufactured results. Furthermore, the author is honest, open and clear about the weaknesses of the results (e.g. the absence of a response from seven education centres and how this may have effected the results/conclusions).

9C Members stated that the author could have made the conclusion clearer. The author does allude to some interesting discussion points (although a thorough critique of the discussion points falls outside of the headings of Burns and Grove's approach). However, members felt that the discussion points would have benefited from further development. Of particular interest was the variation in the course content between sites. The author offers limited explanation for this variation; however, members felt that the author had perhaps missed an opportunity to explore this issue in more detail. It was the hope of the members that future research in this area might follow up these points and ask questions such as: how is current mental health policy and the current research agenda reflected in your course content? Does your course content reflect the specific mental health care needs of your local population and local mental health care workforce? How does the course content reflect the theoretical oreintation of the individual course leaders?

10A Members felt the title reflected the focus of the study and identified the key variables, such as they were.

10B The paper contained an abstract which provided an accurate synopsis of the paper.

10C Members felt that the apparent honesty of the author, both with regard to the limitations and reporting of the study, could be regarded as one of the strengths of the paper, as this honesty was evident throughout the paper.

10D There was no evidence of sexist language.

10E It is reasonable to say that opinion was divided on this matter. Clearly papers that focus on 'specialist' rather than generic issues will be directly applicable to a more narrow audience and therefore perhaps less interesting to the wider audience. As stated previously, members also felt that perhaps the author had missed the opportunity to explore some of the 'big' questions, and this omission thus maybe made the paper less interesting. Nevertheless, opinion was offered that suggested this paper did add something to the knowledge base in this area.

11A/B/C There is no mention of ethical issues in the paper. Members felt this was not a significant limitation given the focus and design of the study. Additionally, the guidelines on the practice of ethics committees in medical research involving human subjects, produced in 1990 and 1996 by the Royal College of Physicians, specify that ethical approval is required for a study when:

(a)   the research involves any NHS clients (past or present)
(b)   the research involves the use of client notes or
(c)   the study was undertaken on NHS premises

Given that the study did not meet these criteria, members felt formal ethical approval was not required.

References

Behi, R. and Nolan, M. (1995) Reliability: consistency and accuracy in measurement. *British Journal of Nursing*, **4**(8), 472–5.

Gamble, C. (1995) The Thorn nurse training initiative. *Nursing Standard*, **9**, 31–4.

Hicks, C. (2004) *Research Methods for Clinical Therapists: Applied Project Design and Analysis*. Churchill Livingstone, Edinburgh.

Kelly, B., Long, A. and McKenna, H. P. (2001) Clinical supervision: personal and professional development or the nursing novelty of the 1990s? In: *Fundamental Themes in Clinical Supervision* (eds. J. R. Cutcliffe, T. Butterworth and B. Proctor), pp. 9–24. Routledge, London.

Norman, I. (1998) The changing emphasis of mental health and learning disability nurse education in the UK and the ideal models of its future development. *Journal of Psychiatric and Mental Health Nursing*, **5**, 41–51.

Parahoo, K. (1997) *Nursing Research: Principles, Process and Issues*. Macmillan, London.

Parkes, T. (1997) Reflections from outside in: my journey into, through and beyond psychiatric nursing. In: *The Mental Health Nurse: Views of Practice and Education* (ed. S. Tilley), pp. 58–72. Blackwell Science, Oxford.

Polit, D. F. and Hungler, B. P. (1997) *Essentials of Nursing Research: Methods, Appraisal and Utilization*, 4th edn. Lippincott, Philadelphia.

Royal College of Physicians (1990) *Guidelines on the Practice of Ethics Committees in Medical Research Involving Human Subjects*. The Royal College of Physicians, London.

Royal College of Physicians (1996) *Guidelines on the Practice of Ethics Committees in Medical Research Involving Human Subjects*. The Royal College of Physicians, London.

Stuppy, D. J. (1998) The FACES pain scale: reliability and validity with mature adults. *Applied Nursing Research*, **11**, 84–9.

White, E. and Brooker, C. (1998) Community Mental Health Nursing: National Surveys. *Mental Health Practice*, **2**(2), 8–16.

Example 4: The NPNR National Journal Club: review from the 11th meeting

The paper reviewed was Fletcher, R. E. (1999) The process of constant observation: perspectives of staff and suicidal patients. *Journal of Psychiatric and Mental Health Nursing*, **6**, 9–14.

Abstract/overview

This paper reports on a study which attempted to explore the perceptions of staff regarding the nursing activity of 'constant observations' of suicidal clients in mental health settings. The paper also attempts to elicit the perceptions of clients and then compare the two. The two categories of nursing interventions – therapeutic and controlling – were identified by both groups. Inconsistencies of the perceptions between the two groups were also noted. The author then discusses and explores the implications of these findings.

1A Feedback comments from the members indicated that the author initially listed three objectives which appeared to be clear. However, further on in the paper, the author changes the stated objectives from 'identifying nurses'/clients' perceptions of the purpose, nature and meaning of constant observations' to 'identifying the perceived purposes, nursing actions and feelings of clients and staff'. Such disparity was felt to confuse matters.

1B As the study used a qualitative design, and thus was not concerned with measuring causal relationships between variables, no key variables are mentioned in the study, and this was regarded as appropriate by the members.

1C Given that the paper claimed to utilise a qualitative, ethnographic research method, it was not necessary to include a formal hypothesis, and therefore the omission of a hypothesis need not be regarded as a flaw.

2A Members stated that the author appeared to be suitably qualified for a study of this type.

2B Comments from the members regarding the literature review were less encouraging with some members expressing a sense of puzzlement. Much of the literature cited by the author appeared to be out of date, which was curious given that a wealth of important and more contemporary material on suicide prevention and the nursing care of suicidal people is available (Busteed and Johnstone, 1983; Mental Health Act Commission and Sainsbury Centre for Mental Health, 1997; Moore, 1998).[1]

2C/D Members raised further questions with respect to the logical sequence, organisation and content of the literature review. For example, there was a question raised about why the review commenced with a reference to risk assessment when this was perhaps outside of the scope or remit of the review. Other members noted that the bulk of the literature reviewed was from the USA, which appeared somewhat inappropriate given that the study was undertaken in the UK. Other members felt that the review perhaps lacked critical reading of the literature and failed to provide a clear picture of how each subsequent study had built upon the findings of the previous work in that substantive area. The literature review did include evidence that indicate the alleged benefits and drawbacks of the experience of being placed on 'constant observations', and offering such a balanced view within the review was thought to be a strength of the paper. Some members stated that the claims that 'constant observations' promote the freedom of the individual needed greater substantiation and evidence.

4A/B Members raised several questions concerning the research design and meth-

---

1 The authors would urge a degree of caution when critiquing the literature review of a paper and, more especially, criticising the paper on the grounds of using 'old' references. It is appropriate to raise this as a criticism if recent research has been omitted, yet to arbitrarily regard findings as lacking meaning and/or significance simply because they are 'old' appears to be an ill-advised action. Seminal works can and should be cited, and describing trends in the research findings over time may necessitate reference to older work.

od. The author described the study as 'ethnography'; however, members could not agree with this description. Ethnographic studies are commonly associated with 'thick description' (Atkinson and Hammersley, 1994; Streubert and Carpenter, 1999; Krumeich et al., 2001), yet such description did not appear to be present in the study. Since, according to Morse and Field (1995), ethnography is always informed by the concept of culture, and thus ethnographers ask: 'In what ways do members of a community actively construct their world?', it would appear reasonable to use an ethnographic method to examine the culture of constant observations on mental health wards. However, qualitative studies that are more concerned with uncovering the meaning of being in the world in certain experiences would perhaps benefit from using a phenomenological method (Heidegger, 1962; Benner and Wrubel, 1989; Walters, 1995; Van Manen, 1997). Consequently, since the author proposed to explore the 'meaning of constant observation' (Fletcher 1999, p. 10), a phenomenological method may have been more appropriate.

4C Members noted that attempts to determine the 'validity' of a qualitative study have been strongly criticised. For example, according to Leininger (1994), this would indicate attempting to judge the credibility of a qualitative design by using criteria designed for quantitative studies. However, the author clearly made some attempt to establish the credibility of his findings, firstly, by drawing on a colleague to sort responses according to operational definitions (although the members pointed out that these definitions were not described), and secondly, by attempting to triangulate the data by obtaining data from the clients. While these endeavours to establish the credibility of the findings should be applauded, it should be noted that there are fundamental epistemological, philosophical and methodological flaws with the methods used by the author.

Firstly, the philosophical underpinnings of quantitative research approaches and qualitative research approaches are very different and such differences have been highlighted many times within the methodological literature (see Denzin and Lincoln, 1994; McKenna, 1997; Cutcliffe and McKenna, 1999). Consequently, key authorities on qualitative research point out that it is inappropriate to attempt to apply positivistic and empiricist views of the world to qualitative research (Morse, 1991a; Denzin and Lincoln, 1994; Ashworth, 1997; Angen, 2000). That the author strives for 'objectivity' within a qualitative study can be regarded as inappropriate.

Members wondered why the author had drawn upon qualitative research texts with a noted 'vintage' and had not made use of the more contemporary qualitative research texts. Perhaps the use of these texts, at least in part, explains the author's inappropriate use of terms developed for establishing the authenticity of quantitative findings. A more current examination of these issues may have highlighted that qualitative research findings should be tested for credibility or accuracy using terms and criteria that have been developed exclusively for this very approach (Hammersley, 1992; Cutcliffe and McKenna, 1999; Angen, 2000; Rolfe, 2006). Indeed, Leininger (1994, p. 114) makes this point most clearly when she states:

we must develop and use criteria that fit the qualitative paradigm, rather than use quantitative criteria for qualitative studies. It is awkward and inappropriate to re-language quantitative terms.

4D On a similar note to 4C, given that the author claimed to be using a qualitative design, it would have been inappropriate to criticise the paper on the grounds of replicability, since this is a criterion developed specifically for use within the quantitative paradigm.

5A/B/C/D Members noted that each of the questions raised in this section appear to be more appropriate for quantitative studies, and should not be criteria for judging the quality of a qualitative piece of research. However, with regard to the congruency between the research design and the data collection method, the use of participant observation within an ethnographic study would have been entirely appropriate (Atkinson and Hammersley, 1994). Therefore this can be regarded as a sound methodological decision within the paper. Perhaps the author could have improved this section of the paper by adding further detail and substantiation to the methodological, data collection decisions he made. For example, what is gained by combining participant observation with interviews? Did the interview schedule evolve or remain static? Were there any questions asked by the participants regarding elements that they felt may have been overlooked?

6A/B Just as in section 5, members noted that each of the questions raised in this section appears to be more appropriate for quantitative studies, and should not be criteria for judging the quality of a qualitative piece of research.

7A Members raised several issues regarding the sampling procedures and felt that they could have been described more clearly. For example, while the composition of the sample was described, unfortunately however, the author provided no explanation of the sampling procedure. Given the relatively small sample size and the qualitative nature of the study, members assumed that the author had used purposeful sampling, which would be in keeping with the method (Morse, 1991b). Yet this was not indicated in the paper. The author included one criterion for inclusion for the sample of clients, though did not include any inclusion criteria for the sample of staff. Members felt that the author should have included an indication of the minimum criteria for inclusion in the sample, thus pointing out what constituted a 'good informant' for this study (Morse, 1991b).

7B/C Given that the author claimed to be using a qualitative design, it would have been inappropriate to criticise the paper on the grounds of the lack of random sampling or the size of the sample. Sampling within qualitative studies is purposefully biased, a point made by Morse (1998, p. 734). She states:

> that means that we seek informants who have experience, *the most experience* [original emphasis] in the topic of interest. Yes, the sample is biased; *it must be biased* [original emphasis].

8A/B/C Given that the author claimed to be using a qualitative design, it would have been inappropriate to criticise the paper on the grounds of the lack of statistical analysis, or the choice of inappropriate statistical tests, or the absence of levels of significance.

9A Members felt that the results did appear to be grounded in the data, and the author substantiated his findings by using text from the interviews, thus adding to the sense that the results were grounded in the data provided by the interviewees.

9B/C Some members stated that the results resonated very clearly with their own experiences and supported themes in this substantive area; namely, the perception of 'constant observations' as a controlling or therapeutic activity (Briggs, 1974; Barker and Walker, 1999; Conway, 1999; Barker and Cutcliffe, 1999; Cutcliffe and Barker, 2002). Other members felt that the results and conclusions could have been explained more clearly.

10A Members felt the title was concise and reflected the area under study.

10B Both the title and the abstract aroused the interest of the members and they stated that the substantive area warranted investigation and study.

10C/E Members found the paper to be interesting and it was particularly refreshing to see such 'honest' data regarding the use and purpose of 'constant observations'. An example of such honesty is the author's finding that acknowledges that, despite the rhetoric of 'supportive observation' (Barker and Cutcliffe, 1999), the use of 'constant observations' clearly has an element of serving the needs of the organisation rather than the needs of the individual. A further strength of the paper, according to the members, was the author's attempt to obtain data, and subsequently induce a theory, from the clients' perspectives. Emotionally charged and sensitive topics within psychiatric/mental health nursing, such as the use of 'constant observations', physical restraint, being detained under the Mental Health Act, or considering a client's sexual needs, each appear to be under-researched. Furthermore, examination of the empirical literature in this area appears to indicate that there is a distinct paucity of research that seeks to elicit the client's perspectives, feelings and experiences of emotionally charged topics. Therefore a study such as this, despite its limitations, might be regarded as a useful contribution to this under-researched substantive area.

10D There was no evidence of sexist language used.

11A/B/C Members stated that there appeared to be no mention of ethical concerns within the study, and such an oversight was regarded as a significant limitation of the study. The members' difficulty can perhaps be located in the concerns regarding research and vulnerable groups. Beauchamp and Childress (1994) reasoned that vulnerable groups are those captive populations, and examples of such populations include the mentally ill, the acutely ill and the terminally ill. Usher and Holmes (1997) argue that vulnerable research participants are those that are considered to be unable, or less able, to make autonomous decisions regarding their participation in the research. According to Watson (1992), when considering whether or not people from these populations should be asked to participate in research studies there are several key factors to consider. The most frequently cited of these factors are the seriousness and probability of risk to the client, whether or not the subject or society receives any benefits, and the capability of the subject to give informed consent. It should be noted that, given the emergent nature of the design of some (most) qualitative studies, it may not always be possible for researchers to balance the benefit to risk ratio of such studies in advance (Raudonis, 1992; Lacey, 1992). However, *ex post facto* consideration of ethical issues or the use of the *ethics as process approach* (Ramcharan and Cutcliffe, 2001; Cutcliffe and Ramcharan, 2002) is more common in social science research, and would have been entirely appropriate for this study.

References

Angen, M. J. (2000) Evaluating interpretive inquiry: reviewing the validity debate and opening the dialogue. *Qualitative Health Research*, **10**(3), 378–95.

Ashworth, P. (1997) The variety of qualitative research: introduction to the problem. *Nurse Education Today*, **17**, 215–18.

Atkinson, P. and Hammersley, M. (1994) Ethnography and participant observation. In: *Handbook of Qualitative Research* (eds. N. K. Denzin and Y. S. Lincoln), pp. 248–61. Sage, London.

Barker, P. and Cutcliffe, J. R. (1999) Clinical risk: a need for engagement not observation. *Mental Health Practice*, **2**(8), 8–12.

Barker, P. and Walker, L. (1999) *A Survey of Care Practices in Acute Admission Wards*. Report submitted to the Northern and Yorkshire Regional Research and Development Committee.

Beauchamp, T. L. and Childress, J. F. (1994) *Principles of Biomedical Ethics*, 4th edn. Oxford University Press, Oxford.

Benner, P. and Wrubel, J. (1989) *The Primacy of Caring: Stress and Coping in Health and Illness*. Addison-Wesley, New York.

Briggs, P. F. (1974) Specialling in psychiatry: therapeutic or custodial? *Nursing Outlook*, **22**, 632–5.

Busteed, E. L. and Johnstone, C. (1983) The development of suicide precautions for in-patient psychiatric units. *Journal of Psychosocial Nursing and Mental Services*, **21**, 15–19.

Conway, E. (1999) *A Multidimensional Audit of Observation Policy*. Report to Newcastle City Health Trust.

Cutcliffe, J. R. and Barker, P. (2002) Considering the care of the suicidal client and the case for 'engagement and inspiring hope' or observations. *Journal of Psychiatric and Mental Health Nursing*. **9**(5), 611–21.

Cutcliffe, J. R. and McKenna, H. P. (1999) Establishing the credibility of qualitative research findings: the plot thickens. *Journal of Advanced Nursing*, **30**(2), 374–80.

Cutcliffe, J. R. and Ramcharan, P. (2002) Levelling the playing field: considering the 'ethics as process' approach for judging qualitative research proposals. *Qualitative Health Research*, **12**(7), 1000–10.

Denzin, N. and Lincoln, Y.S. (1994) Introduction: entering the field of qualitative enquiry. In: *Handbook of Qualitative Research* (eds. N. K. Denzin and Y. S. Lincoln). Sage, London.

Fletcher, R. E. (1999) The process of constant observation: perspectives of staff and suicidal patients. *Journal of Psychiatric and Mental Health Nursing*, **6**, 9–14.

Hammersley, M. (1992) *What's Wrong with Ethnography?* Routledge, London.

Heidegger, M. (1962) *Being and Time*. Harper & Row, New York.

Krumeich, A., Weijts, W., Reddy, P. and Meijer-Weitz, A. (2001) The benefits of anthropological approaches for health promotion research and practice. *Health Education Research*, **16**(2), 121–30.

Lacey, E. A. (1998) Social and medical research ethics: is there a difference? *Social Sciences in Health*. **4**(4), 211–17.

Leininger, M. (1994) Evaluation criteria and critique of qualitative research studies. In: *Critical Issues in Qualitative Research Methods* (ed. J. M. Morse), p. 95–115. Sage, London.

McKenna, H. P. (1997) *Nursing Theories and Models*. Routledge, London.

Mental Health Act Commission and Sainsbury Centre for Mental Health (1997) *The National Visit*. Sainsbury Centre, London.

Moore, C. (1998) Acute in-patient care could do better, says survey. *Nursing Times*, **94**(3), 54–6.

Morse, J. M. (1991a) Qualitative nursing research: a free for all? In: *Qualitative Nursing Research: A Contemporary Dialogue* (ed. J. M. Morse), pp. 14–22. Sage, London.

Morse, J. M. (1991b) Strategies for sampling. In: *Qualitative Nursing Research: A Contemporary Dialogue* (ed. J. M. Morse), pp. 127–45. Sage, London.

Morse, J. M. (1998) What's wrong with random selection? *Qualitative Health Research*. **8**(6), 733–5.

Morse, J. M. and Field, P. A. (1995) *Qualitative Research Methods for Health Professionals*, 2nd edn. Sage, London.

Ramcharan, P. and Cutcliffe, J. R. (2001) Judging the ethics of qualitative research: considering the 'ethics as process' model. *Health and Social Care*, **9**(6), 358–67.

Raudonis, B. M. (1992) Ethical considerations in qualitative research with hospice patients. *Qualitative Health Research*, **2**(2), 238–49.

Rolfe, G. (2006) Judgments without rules: towards a postmodern ironist concept of research validity. *Nursing Inquiry*, **13**, 7–15.

Streubert, H. J. and Carpenter, D. R. (1999) *Qualitative Research in Nursing: Advancing the Humanistic Imperative*, Lippincott, London.

Usher, L. and Holmes, C. (1997) Ethical aspects of phenomenological research with mentally ill people. *Nursing Ethics*, **4**(1), 49–56.

Van Manen, M. (1997) *Researching Lived Experience: Human Science for Action Sensitive Pedagogy*. State University of New York Press, New York.

Walters, A. J. (1995) The phenomenological movement: implications for nursing research. *Journal of Advanced Nursing*, **22**, 791–9.

Watson, A. B. (1992) Informed consent of special subjects. *Nursing Research*, **31**, 43–7.

Summary: strengths and limitations of Burns and Grove's (1985) approach to critiquing nursing research

Strengths

- The approach is easy to follow.
- It does not contain unnecessary jargon and is accordingly accessible.

- The approach leads the reviewer to most of the key components of quantitative studies.
- It is possible that the author of the research paper reviewed may learn from a critique using Burns and Grove's approach, particularly if the reviewers include extensive comments.
- The approach does enable both strengths and limitations to be identified.
- The approach allows room for the data and/or argument to be introduced to support the reviewer's criticisms/observations and suggestions for improvement. However, this relies on the rigour and thoroughness of the reviewer(s), in that the questions asked within the key areas are 'closed questions' i.e. questions that can be adequately answered using single-word responses.

Limitations

- Specifying the need to consider variables (see key area/question 3) shows a limitation of the approach to critiquing, since the absence of variables might not necessarily be indicative of an absence of quality.
- The approach doesn't tell the reviewer all they need to consider in the study. For example, the 'ethics' key area (area 11) asks specific questions about anonymity, confidentiality and informed consent. However, it does not include specific questions about equally important ethical issues, e.g. the balance of risk to benefit ratio.
- A criticism of the Burns and Grove approach is the lack of emphasis on the 'discussion' section and the implications of the results. This is another important example of the approach not informing the reviewer to consider key aspects of a study. In addition to being methodologically sound and having accurate results, studies should also explore, in detail, the implications of these findings. Practitioners need to see the results examined and discussed within the context of current knowledge, conflicting findings and supporting evidence. The absence of a 'discussion' key area within Burns and Grove's approach might then be regarded as a significant omission.
- A further important criticism is the clear emphasis in this approach on critiquing quantitative studies and using quantitative criteria. In fact, we would argue that this approach is unsuitable for critiquing qualitative studies given the focus of the key areas and questions.
- Burns and Grove do not indicate why there are three questions within most of their eleven key areas, four questions in some key areas and two questions in one key area. Thus reviewers might be left wondering if this indicated, implicitly, the relative importance that Burns and Grove ascribe to each of the key areas.

■ This approach, like Duffy's (1985) approach, might be regarded as a form of simplistic reductionism, wherein an attempt is made to reduce the research to its simplest constituent parts, and then the reviewer attempts to 'measure' these parts.[2]

---

2 It should be noted that Burns and Grove perhaps recognised the limitations of their 1987 approach, and subsequently, in later editions of the same book (2nd edn 1993; 3rd edn 1997) they provide more comprehensive approaches, indeed suggesting that quantitative and qualitative studies should be critiqued according to different criteria. However, it is only within the third edition that they include a separate and comprehensive approach for critiquing qualitative studies.

CHAPTER 5

Morrison's (1991) approach to critiquing nursing research

This chapter focuses on Morrison's (1991) approach to critiquing nursing research. Morrison argues that each reader needs to be critical of the research they read in order to discriminate between the high and lower quality papers. Furthermore, he provides a series of reasons for the need to critique research, including the need to 'demystify' research. Morrison then describes what he claims are the five essential features of a critique. He acknowledges that while there any many ways that a reader can critique a study, each of these appears to involve a questioning approach; asking key and/or relevant questions at certain stages of the report. Included in Morrison's approach are questions that he feels need to be asked of the researcher – questions regarding the researcher's knowledge base and depth of background reading. The remainder of his approach is concerned with key questions about the different aspects of the study. Therefore this chapter lists Morrison's key questions under each of the headings he identifies. Following this, we provide two detailed examples (drawing from the reviews carried out by the NPNR Journal Club). Having described the approach and provided examples, we then highlight some of the strengths and limitations of this approach.

Morrison (1991) argues that the central features of a good critique are that the critique should be:

- objective
- constructive
- unbiased
- a penetrating analysis
- a decisive analysis of the quality of the research

Furthermore, the key questions that need to be asked, are grouped under the following headings.

1. Questions about the researcher:
   Who is the researcher and what is his or her background?
2. Questions to ask about the research problem include:
   A Is the problem clearly stated?

    B Can it be easily researched?

    C Has it been researched already or is the researcher providing a new and creative slant?

    D Does the question relate to nursing practice?

3. Questions to ask about the literature review include:

    A Is it relevant to the topic?

    B Is it comprehensive or have key references been ignored or missed out?

    C Are the sources current and up to date or has the author relied solely on well known but out of date references?

    D Is it laid out logically and coherently?

    E Is a summary provided at the end of the review which accurately captures the crucial aspects of the relevant literature and spells out the relevance of this literature for the study?

4. Questions to ask about the design of the study include:

    A Is there a statement about the overall design of the study, such as 'case study', 'experiment' or 'survey', which conveys immediately the type of report which is being discussed?

    B Are the relevant theoretical frameworks discussed?

    C If hypotheses are offered, are they stated clearly?

    D Is there a straightforward description of what the researcher planned to do and why, and how was it done (i.e. aims and methods)?

    E Could we repeat the procedure on the basis of the information provided?

    F Are the technical terms clearly defined or does the author assume that these are understood?

5. Questions to ask about the data collection include:

    A Is the method used discussed in sufficient detail?

    B Is the rationale provided for the choice of method?

    C Does the method stand up to criticism?

    D What details are provided about the sample used in the study?

    E Was the sample appropriate?

    F Are details given about the special instruments used in the study (e.g. questionnaires, interview schedules, measuring techniques)?

    G Is the reliability and validity of the findings discussed?

6. Questions to ask about the data analysis include:

    A Are the analyses appropriate for the type of data collected?

    B Is the method of analysis clearly described, step by step, and easy to follow?

    C Are the findings presented clearly with the help of graphs, tables or highlighted themes?

    D Are the results discussed adequately?

    E Does the discussion emphasise some aspects of the results and ignore others, and is such emphasis justified?

7. Questions to ask about the conclusions and recommendations include:
   A Are the conclusions justified on the strength of the findings?
   B Are the conclusions linked closely to the original purpose of the research?
   C Have any new insights been uncovered during the research?
   D Have new research questions emerged unexpectedly from the study?
   E Are the recommendations made by the researcher feasible and are they excessive and costly?
   F Is a change in nursing practice justified on the strength of these findings or is more research needed before embarking on a programme of major change?
   G What are the implications of the study for further research in the field?
   H Does the researcher evaluate the study and point out possible limitations?

Example 5: The Network for Psychiatric Nursing Research Journal Club: Review from the 15th meeting

The paper reviewed was Allen, J. (1998) A survey of psychiatric nurses' opinions of advanced practice roles in psychiatric nursing. *Journal of Psychiatric and Mental Health Nursing*, **5**, 451–462.

Abstract/overview

In this paper, the author attempted to survey established psychiatric nurses' opinions of the content of advanced practitioner nursing roles by sending a questionnaire to a random sample of 100 members of the NPNR network, and received a response rate of 78%. The results identified elements of the 'normal' nursing roles (e.g. basic psychotherapeutic practices), and elements of the 'advanced' nursing role (e.g. enhanced autonomy in admission and discharge). The study concluded that an advanced psychiatric nursing role was supported by psychiatric nurses and recommended that pilot sites, to test the acceptability and effectiveness of the role, should be established.

I The author is a Registered Mental Nurse (RMN), with a background and current interest in acute psychiatry. He appears to have limited experience of research (assuming that the MSc qualification involved the production of a research dissertation).

2A The author alludes to the research problem early in the paper (second paragraph, Introduction), but members felt that the problem could have been stated more clearly. Later in the paper, the author does indicate a research question; however this occurs at the end of a somewhat discursive section. Members stated that, as a consequence, it was difficult to locate the research question as it was somewhat obscured by the discursive text. Indeed, while acknowledging the need to set the background to the study, members felt that perhaps this section of the paper did not add to the overall clarity of the paper. Furthermore, they added that this section rather confused matters since it gave the paper a 'discursive' appearance rather than an 'empirical' appearance. Thus there may have been merit in condensing this section.

2B The problem can be researched, but members noted that since opinions change over time, any results obtained would need to be acknowledge as a cross-sectional 'snapshot' in time (Polit *et al.*, 2001).

2C The author points out that there is a distinct paucity of empirical work in this area. The author makes reference to some of the theoretical and policy literature in this substantive area, but given the paucity of empirical work, particularly exploration of psychiatric nurses' views of advanced practice, the research has the potential to be contributing new knowledge.

2D Members felt that the research question clearly relates directly to nursing practice and, potentially, could relate to psychiatric nursing education, policy and further research.

3A Members noted that the paper does not include an identified literature review. There appeared to be no systematic or logical review of the previous studies undertaken in this substantive area.

3B The author does include a review of some of the theoretical literature (e.g. the arguments regarding specialist or advanced, extended or expanded practice) and draws upon additional literature which may be related to this substantive area (e.g. nurse prescribing). However, as stated previously, members stated that while this did allude to the background of the study in part, it retained a discursive feel and did not appear to provide a comprehensive review of all the research in this area. Having said that, it may be that such texts do not currently exist within the British literature. Nevertheless, given that the author drew upon North American theoretical texts, it might have been prudent for the author to review the empirical work that also originated from America.

3C The sources used are current, but as stated previously, the sources are primarily from theoretical and policy literature, not from empirical work.

3D Members felt that this section of the paper was perhaps somewhat confusing as they wished to see a review of the empirical work carried out in this area in order that they could see the current extent of the knowledge base in this substantive area.

3E There did not appear to be a summary at the end of the review which accurately captured the crucial aspects of the relevant literature.

4A The paper does include a statement that suggests that the research design used a postal survey. However, members pointed out that this statement was misleading. Further into the paper (p. 455), the author points out that the study included a qualitative analysis. Therefore, to describe the research design as using only a survey could be regarded as inaccurate, and it might have been more accurate to describe the study as using a triangulated design (Nolan and Behi, 1995; Fu-Jin, 1998; Polit *et al.*, 2001).

4B The author includes some information on the survey design, but members still raised some questions over this matter. Firstly, they felt that some justification for the use of a survey might have enhanced the quality of the paper. Particularly, when arguments about the longitudinal and cumulative nature of knowledge generation are considered (Popper, 1965; May, 1994; McKenna, 1997). Additionally, the members recognise the inclusion of some operationally defined terms regarding 'normal, generalist, and specialist' practice, and they felt such definitions were a strength of the paper. However, they did wonder if the respondents had been provided with these terms, since their own understanding of these terms might have been different from the author's. Such differences may not necessarily invalidate the results, but members felt it might have been useful to know if all the respondents were responding to the same conceptualisations of different 'levels' of practice.

4C No hypotheses were used.

4D The paper included some information regarding the description of the study, but as stated previously, perhaps could have included more. Members suggested, for example, some rationale for using what the author refers to as 'qualitative data', and how this would address the aims of the study.

4E Members felt there was enough information to enable a repeat of the study, although they added that they would clarify and enhance the 'qualitative' component before repeating this study.

4F The feedback from the members indicated that they felt that, on the whole, the technical terms had been clearly defined.

5A The method used was described.

5B As stated previously, the author could have explained his justification for using a survey in more detail.

5C Members noted that the author claimed to have undertaken a qualitative analysis of the comments written in response to the questions, and they went on to level strong criticisms of this section of the paper. Firstly, the members noted that there is no description later in the paper of the 'themes' the author claimed he would introduce. Perhaps more importantly, members questioned whether or not the author had undertaken what could be accurately described as qualitative research at all.

Whilst acknowledging the many forms of qualitative research, both Morse (1991) and Cutcliffe (1997) point out that many studies that purport to be using a qualitative method are arguably not doing so. In this paper, there does not appear to be any evidence of analysis, or evidence of the analytical processes required in qualitative research. Counting the same word or phrase, contained in the additional 'comments' in response to deductive questions, such as the author has in this paper, does not constitute qualitative data analysis. Qualitative researchers need repeated and in-depth contact with their data. This is often expressed in terms of 'immersing oneself in the data' (Streubert and Carpenter, 1999) and it is this repeated contact which enables them to witness re-occurring patterns and themes in the data: qualitative researchers are not concerned with searching for the same word or phrase. Indeed, awkward attempts to count the frequency of the same word in qualitative data analysis have been strongly criticised as inappropriate. Morse (1995, p. 148) makes this point most clearly when she states:

> I repeat: The **quantity** [original emphasis] of data in a category is not theoretically important to the process of saturation. Richness of data derived from detailed description, not the number of times something is stated. Frequency counts are out.

Additionally (p. 147):

> Frequency of occurrence of any specific incident must be ignored. Saturation involves eliciting all forms of types of occurrences, valuing variation over quantity.

5D Members felt that the size of the sample appeared to be adequate for a preliminary study, although they noted the absence of power calculations (Cohen, 1977; Peat, 2002; Hicks, 2004). Power calculations or 'power analysis' can be carried out in order to determine how large the sample needs to be (by using an estimation of the size of the difference expected between two groups). Questions were raised about the representativeness of the sample as it was taken from the NPNR members. However, the author did acknowledge this as a limitation of the study.

5E Parts of the questionnaire were described in detail, including some operational definitions.

5F Unfortunately, the paper contains no reference to reliability or validity, and this was thought to be a significant omission. It may have been particularly valuable and prudent to use a 'test/re-test' design in order to establish the reliability of the instrument (Behi and Nolan, 1995; Parahoo, 1997; Peat, 2002; Hicks, 2004), particularly as the study was concerned with measuring opinion, and it is well accepted that opinions change over time.

6A The members raised several issues with regard to the choice and the use of the statistical tests of the author. According to Watson and McFadyen's (1997) paper on non-parametric tests (*note: one of these authors is a senior lecturer in statistics*), it would have been more appropriate to use the Wilcoxon signed rank test to determine statistical significance differences within the single sample, rather than the

Mann–Whitney U-test, which is most often associated with testing for significant differences between two independent samples. Perhaps it could argued that the author achieved two independent samples (i.e. practice-based and academic staff). However, the author states that he selected a random sample of 100 NPNR members and thus does not appear to have purposefully selected independent samples. Furthermore, given that Chi-square tests are usually undertaken to determine statistical significance associations between two categorical scales (Watson and McFaden, 1997), it was unclear which two categorical scales the author was referring to in his paper.

6B There was mixed opinion in response to this question; some members felt that the methods of analysis were adequately described, whereas other members thought they were confusing. For example, members wondered whether it was legitimate to manipulate/remove the results (see p. 456) and how this manipulation might have affected the results.

6C Opinion was mixed on this matter. Some members felt that the methods of analysis were adequately described; others thought that they were confusing and could have been made clearer. Possibly the use of percentages would have helped. Furthermore, the jumps in the item question numbers (e.g. 1.1, then 12.4, then 14.1) were rather confusing.

6D Again, opinion was mixed on this matter, but on the whole, the members felt that the results could have been described more clearly. They raised a particular concern over the use of the term 'a high level of comments' (p. 459), as this indicated evidence of confusion of and combining qualitative and quantitative methods in an inappropriate manner (Cutcliffe and McKenna, 1999).

6E The discussion appears to offer a balanced argument, and an argument that arises out of the findings. However, given the paucity of the research in this area, and the disparity of the nature of advanced practice evident within the results, perhaps a more appropriate study to undertake would have been to ask: what activities should 'normal, advanced and specialist' psychiatric nursing practice be composed of?

7A Members felt that the conclusions were partially justified by the results. However, given the methodological limitations, the possible unrepresentative nature of the sample, the absence of any reliability or validity measures, and the cross-sectional nature of the study, it might have been more appropriate for the author to phrase his conclusion in a tentative manner, rather than the 'assertive' manner used in the paper.

7B Members stated that the conclusions are linked closely to the original purpose of the research.

7C Members stated that whilst the research did not uncover any new insights with this research, the findings did reiterate theoretical (and valuable) positions, in particular the importance of ensuring that advanced nursing roles do not become a 'dumping ground' for practices no longer desired by medics.

7D The author mentions the need for future additional surveys, with different and wider professions; however, no new research questions were identified and the members felt this was a notable omission.

7E Members felt that the practice and educational recommendations posited by the author were feasible, but as with any new training initiative, they would have an additional cost attached.

7F Members felt that far more research was required before it would reasonable to justify major changes in nursing practice/service delivery.

7G Members felt that the paper highlighted additional lines of enquiry and the need for further research. Perhaps studies could be conducted with psychiatric nurses who work in different clinical areas. Additional surveys with larger and more representative samples might be worthwhile. But perhaps more importantly, this study would lead to studies that ask related questions, but questions more appropriate to the current extent of knowledge in this substantive area (see 6E).

7H The author does point out some of the limitations of the study, but perhaps it would have been prudent to acknowledge more of them (e.g. absence of reliability/validity measures, methodological limitations).

References

Behi, R. and Nolan, M. (1995) Reliability: consistency and accuracy in measurement. *British Journal of Nursing*, **4**(8), 472–5.

Cohen, J. (1977) *Statistical Power Analysis for the Behavioral Sciences* (rev. edn). Academic Press, New York.

Cutcliffe, J. R. (1997) Qualitative research in nursing: a quest for quality. *British Journal of Nursing*, **6**(17), 969.

Cutcliffe, J. R. and McKenna, H. P. (1999) Establishing the credibility of qualitative research findings: the plot thickens. *Journal of Advanced Nursing*, **30**(2), 374–80.

Fu-Jin, S. (1998) Triangulation in nursing research: issues of conceptual clarity and purpose. *Journal of Advanced Nursing*, **28**(3), 631–41.

Hicks, C. (2004) *Research Methods for Clinical Therapists: Applied Project Design and Analysis.* Churchill Livingstone, Edinburgh.

May, K. A. (1994) Abstract knowing: the case for magic in the method. In: *Critical Issues in Qualitative Research Methods* (ed. J. M. Morse), pp. 10–21. Sage, London.

McKenna, H. P. (1997) *Nursing Theories and Models.* Routledge, London.

Morse, J. M. (1991) Qualitative nursing research: a free-for-all? In: *Qualitative Nursing Research: A Contemporary Dialogue* (ed. J. M. Morse), pp. 14–22. Sage, London.

Morse, J. M. (1995) The significance of saturation. *Qualitative Health Research*, **5**(2), 147–9.

Nolan, M. and Behi, R. (1995) Triangulation: the best of all worlds? *British Journal of Nursing*, **4**(14), 829–32.

Parahoo, K. (1997) *Nursing Research: Principles, Process and Issues.* Macmillan, London.

Peat, J. (with Mellis, C., Williams, K. and Xuan, W.) (2002) *Health Science Research: A Handbook of Quantitative Methods.* Sage, London.

Polit, D. F., Beck, C. T. and Hungler, B. P. (2001) *Essentials of Nursing Research: Methods, Appraisal and Utilization*, 5th edn. Lippincott, Philadelphia.

Popper, K. (1965) *Conjectures and Refutations: the Growth of Scientific Knowledge*. Harper & Row, New York.

Streubert, H. J. and Carpenter, D. R. (1999) *Qualitative Research in Nursing: Advancing the Humanistic Imperative*, 2nd edn. Lippincott, Philadelphia

Watson, H. and McFadyen, A. (1997) Nonparametric analysis. *Nurse Researcher*, **4**(4), 28–40.

Example 6: The NPNR National Journal Club: Review from the 8th meeting

The paper reviewed was Pejlert, A., Asplund, K., Gilje, F. and Norberg, A. (1998) The meaning of caring for patients on a long-term psychiatric ward as narrated by formal care providers. *Journal of Psychiatric and Mental Health Nursing*, **5**, 255–64.

Abstract/overview

This paper reports on a study that interviewed 17 care providers about their caring experiences on a hospital psychiatric ward, and attempted to elicit the meaning of this work. The study used Ricoeur's (1976) phenomenological hermeneutic method and induced three themes which illuminated the meaning of care provided. These were described as: being in the midst of human storage; moving towards a human care of relations; and struggling with the old and the new. The authors then interpreted and discussed these findings in the light of a previously published interview study, one which obtained the experiences of the patients who lived on a long-term psychiatric ward. The authors conclude that attending to ingrained attitudes of the past and their influence on the new approaches to care is essential to understanding not only changes in ways of doing nursing tasks, but also ways of relating.

1 From the qualifications of the authors, it appeared as though the authors represented a collection of nurse educators from several academic centres, some of whom appeared to have a clinical background. It was unclear from these qualifications precisely what the nature of this clinical background might have been.

2A Members felt that the research question was not clearly stated. Indeed, they added that while the title appears to be clear, it does not accurately reflect the content of the paper. It should be noted that the introduction creates more confusion around the nature of the study. While the title indicates that the study is concerned with eliciting the meaning of caring for long-term psychiatric patients, the introduction claims that the study aims to elicit the narratives of patients as well as carers. Consequently, members thought that the paper could have made the research question clearer.

2B Members stated that they had difficulty answering this point, since they were unclear what 'easily researched' means. However, exploring or attempting to understand the meanings that people ascribe to their lived experiences or basic social processes is entirely appropriate (and plausible) for a qualitative study (Glaser and

Strauss, 1967; Van Manen, 1997; Streubert and Carpenter, 1999). Therefore it is reasonable to argue that the problem can be researched (although whether or not this is 'easy' is another matter.)

2C It was noted that the introduction consists largely of a detailed account of a previous, but linked, study conducted by the same authors, and a review of some other studies that appear to be linked to this substantive area. However, while there appears to exist a limited body of work in this (or related) substantive areas, members posited that there appeared to be a paucity of empirical work focused on this research issue with this particular client population. Consequently, the paper had the potential to add something new to the formal area of 'caring'.

2D The problem clearly relates to nursing practice. Indeed, it claimed to be a study concerned with understanding the very nature of nursing practice for a specific population.

3A Members stated that it appeared that the introduction and literature review were blurred. Additionally, it might be regarded as inappropriate to have such a detailed account of the previous study at this point in the paper. However, it would seem appropriate and relevant to cite the previous studies of the authors and thereby highlight an ongoing theme or context to their research.

3B/C The literature review appeared to contain few references; however, given that the authors claimed to be using a qualitative method, it could be argued as inappropriate to carry out a comprehensive literature review at this point (see Glaser and Strauss, 1967). However, if this limited reviewing of the literature was a purposeful and necessary component of the method, the authors do not make this clear. Furthermore, they appear to allude (briefly) to the theoretical literature and limited empirical literature in this substantive area (i.e. experiences of 'caring' for mental health clients). Therefore members were unsure if this was a purposeful and necessary component of the method or evidence of an incomplete literature review.

3D As stated above, the sequence and layout were regarded as rather confusing, since the author appeared to have combined the introduction and the literature review, and the members questioned the inclusion of so much detail from the authors' previous study.

3E There was no evidence of a summary of the main points of the literature review.

4A There did not appear to be a statement about the overall design of the study. The methods section was subdivided into four sub-sections: participants and setting, interviews, interpretation and results, and naïve reading. Questions raised by the members included the inquiry if each of these sub-sections was appropriate to the methods section of the study. The first sub-section – participants and setting – says very little about the methods but does include detailed information on the participants.

4B There did not appear to be a discussion of the relevant theoretical frameworks.

4C The paper did not appear to contain any stated hypotheses. However, given that the authors claimed to be using a qualitative method, it could be argued that a formal hypothesis was not required (see Glaser, 1978). Bearing in mind that a hypothesis refers to a proposed relationship between variables, and this study was concerned with examining the 'meanings' of caring for a certain client group, the absence of a formal hypothesis was not felt to be a limitation of the study. Rather, it was a methodological choice that was congruent with the design.

4D Members felt that while the paper contained one sentence which described the aims of the study (within the introduction, p. 257), the methods and sub-sections were rather confusing. Members noted how the authors claimed that they asked three questions in the interview. Yet in this section alone there are at least five questions. Unfortunately, there is no indication of the actual nature of these questions, but if this is an example of the multiplicity of the questions used, members felt it raised doubts about the ability of the authors to identify appropriately matched responses. Members wondered: if the questions and responses do not link, how could the data be coded correctly?

4E Once again, given that the study claimed to be using a qualitative method, and that qualitative approaches are not concerned with establishing reliability by the use of replication (Morse and Field, 1995; Rolfe, 2006), members felt it would have been inappropriate to criticise this study on the grounds of it lacking the necessary information to make replication possible.

4F The members did not raise the over-use of technical 'jargon' as an issue for this text; they were, however, of the opinion that the structure and the arrangement of the information contained in the paper was somewhat equivocal and confusing. Furthermore, they felt that the paper contained too much tautological and unnecessary text, and as a result this text might detract from the overall message of the paper.

5A As stated above (in 4D), the section titled 'interviews' appeared to include sufficient detail, yet further reading of the paper indicated contradictions and inconsistencies with this information.

5B The paper does not appear to contain a rationale for the method chosen.

5C The method of data collection (i.e. interviews) was felt to be congruent with the research design (Morse and Field, 1995; Streubert and Carpenter, 1999).

5D The paper contained a wealth of information regarding the characteristics of the sample. However, members pointed out that there did not appear to be any indication of the sampling strategy. At the very least, it would have strengthened the paper if the authors stated they had used a sampling strategy that is in keeping with the research design, i.e. purposeful sampling.

5E Given that all 17 care providers from the particular hospital ward were inter-viewed, members felt that this was an appropriate and adequate sample for this study.

5F As stated above (in 4D/5A), the section titled 'interviews' appeared to include sufficient detail, yet further reading of the paper indicated contradictions and incon-sistencies with this information.

5G Given that this claimed to be a qualitative study, members noted that the ab-sence of validity and reliability measures need not be construed as a limitation. But what would be expected to be present is some attempt or attention to establishing the credibility or authenticity of the findings, and this would be in keeping with quali-tative methods (Leininger, 1992; Cutcliffe and McKenna, 2002). In response to this, members raised some questions concerning the authors' attempts to establish the credibility of their findings by 'checking with a colleague'. There are benefits to this process, in that it provides the opportunity to challenge the robustness of the emerg-ing themes. For instance, there may be issues or patterns that the researcher has missed which the colleague may highlight. It should also be noted that this approach has several philosophical and epistemological difficulties (Cutcliffe and McKenna, 1999). Firstly, since the process of theory induction and the subsequent generation of themes depends upon the unique creative processes between the researcher and the data, it is unlikely that two people will interpret the data in the same way. Second-ly, enlisting the help of a colleague to 'check' or verify the induced themes somehow suggests that if more than one person agrees with the induced themes then this must be more accurate than one person's induction. If this argument is expanded, it begins to support the positivistic philosophy that there is only one accurate interpretation – only one reality – and the accuracy of an interpretation is increased as the number of people agreeing increases.

6A/B Members described the method of data analysis as being congruent with a qualitative design. However, it is reasonable to suggest that they also identified some problems. Members indicated that the third sub-section, 'Interpretation and results', did include the description of the method of data analysis used, but unfortunately did not adequately illustrate how the analysis or interpretation occurred. It did contain a brief explanation of the stages involved in the analysis, but perhaps this section could have been strengthened considerably by providing an example of how a particular theme was induced from the three-stage process described. This might have en-hanced the understanding and explanation of the process and added some credibility to the theory, in that the reader would be able to see the evolution of the theory from the transcripts of the lived experiences of the interviews.

The authors state that the interviewees' texts were read with the pre-understand-ing of the results of their previous study (p. 257). Arguments exist in the qualitative research literature that would appear to support such disclosure. Lincoln and Guba (1985) wrote of neutrality, where researchers can minimise their subjectivity and thus increase the credibility of their findings. This position is based upon the notion that the researcher's previous 'theoretical baggage' would influence unduly the interpretations of the findings. Other authors (e.g. Husserl, 1964; Rose **et al.**, 1995; Jasper, 1994) describe this process as 'bracketing'. They argue that one's experience, judgement and beliefs can be bracketed to avoid these perceptions effecting the findings. Similarly, Ashworth (1993, 1997) holds the view that the credibility of the findings is increased if researchers first make explicit their pre-suppositions and acknowledge their subjective judgement.

A vigorous counter-argument to this position exists. Morse (1994) contends that qualitative methods have been plagued with conflicting advice concerning the application of prior knowledge. Many qualitative authors (Benner, 1984; Benner and Wrubel, 1989; Schutz, 1994; Walters, 1995; Angen, 2000; Cutcliffe, 2003) describe the creativity and interpretation that researchers bring to the study, and that this interpretation can be made richer by immersing all of themselves in the subject's world. Turner (1981) and Stern (1994) posit that it is the reflexivity and researcher's creativity that make qualitative methods so valuable, and Cutcliffe (2003) argues that to deny a qualitative researcher's access to their prior knowledge and restrict the creativity necessary to utilise it is likely to limit the depth of understanding of the phenomenon and impose unnecessary rigid structures. However, the authors of the reviewed paper decided to disclose one particular pre-understanding and this led the members to ask the questions: why disclose only this pre-understanding and not any other pre-understandings that they have? Are the authors suggesting this is the only pre-understanding they have?

6C The paper appears to report and explain its findings under the headings: structural analysis, content, form, interpreted whole and reflection. Members stated that this section contains some limited explanation of the process of analysis, and this improves the overall quality of the paper. Additionally, this section does explain each of the induced themes and the members stated that they could see how the lived experiences and subsequent data had been analysed to form the themes. This section was also felt to be rather repetitive.

6D/E The paper states that the results of the analysis of the data from the care givers (new data) will be presented with the results of the patients' analysis (old data). Members declared that the end product was, realistically, more about the old data than the new. Subsequently, this was felt to be somewhat deceptive and detracted from the overall quality of the paper, as it confused rather than enlightened members. This was felt to be unfortunate, since the group members thought that there were some interesting points and findings in this section, but that they were often obscured and difficult to 'dig out'. There was a great deal of material presented by the authors, and members felt that this was perhaps too much. For example, the paper included a table which took up a whole page of the journal. Perhaps the authors could have condensed this to reflect the key points, or provide examples, and consequently maybe make the paper more 'punchy'. A significant point raised by the members was that, once again, a study that sought to uncover the opinions or experiences of recipients of mental health care found that nurses who were 'kind' and understanding were equated with providing 'good' care.

7A/B Members pointed out that it was difficult to answer this question as the authors had not included or identified a specific 'Conclusions' section within the manuscript.

7C/D Feedback from the group members suggested they felt this was an interesting paper, which at times raised some important questions about the nature of care giver relationships with clients. In particular, it highlighted the shift in emphasis in nursing from the role of 'care giver' to a 'partner in a therapeutic alliance'. These findings reflect a re-occurring theme within current psychiatric and mental health nursing literature: that of the centrality and value of forming relationships with clients and engaging in human care (Barker, 1999). While for some mental health nurses there appears to be a current emphasis on cure, neuroscience and biological interventions, it is important to note that for many others this is regarded as entirely inappropriate. This paper can thus be seen to be adding to the argument that many psychiatric and mental health nurses are becoming increasingly aware of the need to remind themselves of several key questions, such as: what do people need psychiatric or mental health nurses for? How can these nurses establish the genuinely, collaborative forms of care or partnerships, described in the 1994 Report of the Mental Health Review Team (Department of Health 1994)? How can we develop a technology of human care which is undeniably about P/MH nursing? (Barker, 1999).

7E The paper did not appear to contain any recommendations.

7F Members felt that it would be unwise to instigate a change in practice on the grounds of the findings of one study. However, this is not necessarily a reflection on the quality of this paper, but is more indicative of applying an appropriate level of caution when interpreting and subsequently implementing any research findings.

7G As stated above (7 C/D), the findings in this study perhaps indicate the need to undertake empirical work in order to address certain key questions, such as: what do people need P/MH nurses for? How can these nurses establish the genuinely, collaborative forms of care or partnerships, described in the 1994 Report of the Mental Health Review Team (Department of Health 1994)? How can we develop a technology of human care which is undeniably about P/MH nursing (Barker 1999)?

7H The authors do not appear to have included a 'Limitations of the study' section, or indicated the possible limitations in the study. The members thought this was a significant oversight.

References

Angen, M. J. (2000) Evaluating interpretive inquiry: reviewing the validity debate and opening the dialogue. *Qualitative Health Research*, **10**(3), 378–95.

Ashworth, P. D. (1993) Participant agreement in the justification of qualitative findings. *Journal of Phenomenological Psychology*, **25**, 3–16.

Ashworth, P. D. (1997) The variety of qualitative research: non-positivist approaches. *Nurse Education Today*, **17**, 219–24.

Barker, P. (1999) *The Philosophy and Practice of Psychiatric Nursing*. Churchill Livingstone, Edinburgh.

Benner, P. (1984) *From Novice to Expert: Excellence and Power in Clinical Practice*. Addison-Wesley, New York.

Benner, P. and Wrubel, J. (1989) *The Primacy of Caring: Stress and Coping in Health and Illness*. Addison-Wesley, New York.

Cutcliffe, J. R. (2003) Re-considering reflexivity: the case for intellectual entrepreneurship. *Qualitative Health Research*, **13**(1), 136–48.

Cutcliffe, J. R. and McKenna, H. P. (1999) Establishing the credibility of qualitative research findings: the plot thickens. *Journal of Advanced Nursing*, **30**(2), 374–80.

Cutcliffe, J. R. and McKenna, H. P. (2002) When do we know that we know?: considering the truth of research findings and the craft of qualitative research. *International Journal of Nursing Studies*, **39**(6), 611–18.

Department of Health (1994) *Working in Partnership: A Collaborative Approach to Care*. Report of the Mental Health Nursing Review Team. HMSO, London.

Glaser, B. G. (1978) *Theoretical Sensitivity*. Sociology Press, Mill Valley, CA.

Glaser, B. G. and Strauss, A. L. (1967) *The Discovery of Grounded Theory: Strategies for Qualitative Research*, Aldine, Chicago.

Husserl, E. (1964) *The Idea of Phenomenology* (transl. W. Alston and G. Nakhikan). Nijhoff, The Hague.

Jasper, M. A. (1994) Issues in phenomenology for researchers in nursing. *Journal of Advanced Nursing*, **19**, 309–14.

Leininger, M. (1992) Current issues, problems and trends to advanced qualitative paradigmatic research methods for the future. *Qualitative Health Research*, **2**(4), 392–415.

Lincoln, Y. S. and Guba, E. G. (1985) *Naturalistic Enquiry*. Sage, Newbury Park.

Morrison, P. (1991) Critiquing research. *Surgical Nurse*, **4**(3), 20–2.

Morse, J. M. (1994) Emerging from the data: the cognitive processes of analysis in qualitative enquiry. In: *Critical Issues in Qualitative Research Methods* (ed. J. M. Morse), pp. 23–43. Sage, London.

Morse, J. M. and Field, P. A. (1995) *Qualitative Research Methods for Health Professionals*, 2nd edn. Sage, London.

Rolfe, G. (2006) Judgments without rules: towards a postmodern ironist concept of research validity. *Nursing Inquiry*, **13**, 7–15.

Rose, P., Beeby, J. and Parker, D. (1995) Academic rigour in the lived experience of researchers using phenomenological methods in nursing. *Journal of Advanced Nursing*, **21**, 1123–9.

Schutz, S. E. (1994) Exploring the benefits of a subjective approach in qualitative nursing. *Journal of Advanced Nursing*, **20**, 412–17.

Stern, P. (1994) Eroding grounded theory. In: *Critical Issues in Qualitative Research* (ed. J. M. Morse), pp. 210–23. Sage, London.

Streubert, H. J. and Carpenter, D. R. (1999) *Qualitative Research in Nursing: Advancing the Humanistic Imperative*. Lippincott, Philadelphia.

Turner, B. (1981) Some practical aspects of qualitative data analysis: one way of organising the cognitive processes associated with the generation of grounded theory. *Quality and Control*, **15**, 225–45.

Van Manen, M. (1997) *Researching Lived Experience: Human Science for Action Sensitive Pedagogy*. State University of New York Press, New York.

Walters, A. J. (1995) The phenomenological movement: implications for nursing research. *Journal of Advanced Nursing*, **22**, 791–9.

Summary: strengths and limitations of Morrison's approach

Strengths

- The approach is easy to follow and apply.
- It follows a logical sequence that usually matches that of the reviewed paper.
- It appears to give consideration to most of the fundamental components that each research report should make reference to.
- It does not contain an overuse of terminology or jargon, but requires the reviewer to have some understanding of basic concepts and practices within research.
- It is possible that the author of the research paper reviewed may learn from a critique using Morrison's approach, particularly if the reviewers include extensive comments.
- The approach does enable both strengths and limitations to be identified.
- The approach clearly encourages the reviewer(s) to think about how the findings in the reviewed paper(s) may impact on nursing practice. Indeed, the reviewers are encouraged to place the findings in the overall context of the substantive/formal area researched, and that is a notable strength of the approach.
- The approach does include some useful and thought-provoking questions within the headings; for example, question 6E: 'Does the discussion emphasise some aspects of the results and ignore others, and is this emphasis justified?'.
- The approach allows room for the data and/or argument to be introduced to support the reviewer's criticisms/observations and suggestions for improvement. Furthermore, this is perhaps facilitated more easily using Morrison's approach than with the two previous approaches (Duffy, 1985; Burns and Grove, 1993). This is because some of the questions used in Morrison's approach use 'open-ended' rather than closed questions, and thus stimulate more than comments/debate.

Limitations of this approach

- Some of the terminology used in Morrison's questions, or the meaning of the questions, is unclear and thus difficult to assess. For example, what does the author mean by the expression 'easily researched?'. How should a reviewer determine whether or not something is 'easily researched?'. Just because something may be difficult to research, does that make a study any less valuable or appropriate?

■ This approach appears to be more focused on critiquing quantitative studies (e.g. questions about hypotheses, questions about replication of the study, the question about graphs and tables). Consequently, the usefulness of this approach in critiquing qualitative studies may be limited.

■ There are several questions that need to be asked of each reviewed paper which this approach does not indicate or facilitate the reviewer in asking (e.g. the approach makes no reference to ethical issues or ethical considerations).

■ The approach suggests the reviewer should consider whether a change in practice is required as a result of the findings. However, since it would be unwise to instigate a change in practice on the grounds of the findings of one study, this seams like a superfluous question.

■ One of Morrison's questions (3C) asks, 'are the sources [of literature] current and up to date or has the author relied solely on well known but out of date references?'. There are several limitations arising out of this question (even ignoring the tautology). Firstly, Morrison does not indicate when a paper would become 'out of date'. Secondly, and this issue is of greater importance, what reviewers should be considering is the quality of the references included, not necessarily the age. Age as the sole criterion does not always indicate poor quality. Indeed, prudent researchers usually make reference to seminal or key works. Thus, it is difficult to imagine a physics researcher being criticised for including the work of Newton, Faraday or Einstein. Similarly, it would be inappropriate to criticise the work of a researcher examining issues within psychodynamic therapy for including the work of Freud, Klein or Jung.

■ As with Burns and Grove's approach, Morrison does not appear to indicate why there are different numbers of questions within the key areas he identifies. Indeed, the range of the number of questions is wider than in Burns and Grove's approach. Morrison's approach has a key area with one question, some key areas with four questions and even one key area with eight questions! Thus reviewers were left wondering whether this indicated, implicitly, the relative importance that Morrison ascribes to each of the key areas.

■ This approach, like Duffy's (1985) approach and Burns and Grove's (1993) approach might be regarded as a form of simplistic reductionism, wherein an attempt is made to reduce the research to its simplest constituent parts, and then the reviewer attempts to 'measure' these parts.

References

Burns, N. and Grove, S. K. (1993) *The Practice of Nursing Rexearch: Conduct, Critique and Utilization*, 2nd edn. W. B. Saunders, Philadelphia.

Morrison, P. (1991) Critiquing research. *Surgical Nurse*, **4**(3), 20–2.

Ricoeur, P. (1976) *Interpretation Theory: Discourse and the Surplus of Meaning*. Christian University Press, Fort Worth, TX.

Duffy, M. (1985) A research appraisal checklist for evaluating nursing research reports. *Nursing and Healthcare*, **6**(10), 539–47.

CHAPTER 6

Ryan-Wenger's (1992) guidelines for critique of a research report

This chapter focuses on Ryan-Wenger's (1992) guidelines for critiquing nursing research. Ryan-Wenger purports that before the findings reported in a research paper can be used to change clinical practice, the research should first be evaluated for evidence of credibility. It is perhaps notable that some of the language used by Ryan-Wenger (e.g. 'credibility', 'evaluated') is dissimilar to that used in other approaches to critique. Nevertheless, the author strongly asserts that there are three characteristics that will influence the likelihood of publication of a research report: (a) the credibility of the research report, (b) the integrity of the research method, and (c) replication of the research (findings). Ryan-Wenger (1992, p. 394) makes further (perhaps somewhat assertive) comments suggesting that:

> a critique is an objective evaluation of the quality of the written report of an article, the strength of the research design and the adequacy of the author's interpretation of the findings

Whereas some of the other approaches do not make the claim that critique refers to certain accepted standards of research (see for example Polit and Hungler, 1997, discussed in Chapter 7), Ryan-Wenger does, predicating that critique is synonymous with evaluation and that evaluation implies a comparison against accepted standards. In the case of the deductive designs that Ryan-Wenger focuses on, this means comparison against standards derived from (p. 394):

> the tenets of the scientific method

Interestingly, while the title of Ryan-Wenger's paper does not make any distinction between different research paradigms, Ryan-Wenger later declared that her paper is not in any way concerned with critiquing or 'evaluating' studies that use a qualitative design.

Ryan-Wenger describes a two-stage process of critiquing where firstly, the reader is urged to undertake a quick (and objective) overall read of the paper in order to gain a perspective of what was done, why and how it was done.

The second stage appears to involve a more in-depth second read. In order to 'evaluate' the credibility of the research paper Ryan-Wenger urges the reader to examine the five following issues:

1. **Writing style** – according to the author, a well-written report is logically organised and leaves few questions in the mind of the reviewer, thus enhancing the credibility of the report.
2. **Authors** – the author predicates that one can infer credibility on the research findings as a result of the inclusion of brief biographical information (the authors of this book note that this is in and of itself, debatable). Congruence between clinical focus/area of study, having a doctorate level qualification, and previously published work is evidence of enhanced credibility.
3. **Title of the research report** – in this section, Ryan-Wenger argues that certain words/terms can be used to enhance the credibility of the study, whereas she purports that 'catchy' or 'innovative' titles detract from the quality of the work (the authors of this book note that this is also highly debatable).
4. **Abstract** – according to the author, an abstract is credible if it answers (briefly and accurately), why (the problem), who (the sample), what (major variables), why (research hypothesis), how (method), so what (results/discussions) and what now (implications).
5. **Problem** – as with other sections, Ryan-Wenger (1992, p. 395) is somewhat prescriptive about what information to include and where to include it (even suggesting that the research problem should be clearly described in the first paragraph of the report!). The author also declares that quotations from classic or current literature, provocative case examples or poems should not be included as they are 'distracting and detract from the scientific nature of the research'.

In order to 'evaluate' the integrity of the research method Ryan-Wenger urges the reader to examine the following 12 issues:

1. **Logical consistency** – reviewers should attempt to evaluate the congruence between the theoretical framework, review of literature, purpose, research questions, designs, operational definitions, analysis and interpretation of findings.
2. **Theoretical framework** – the author emphasises that deductive research must be based on some theoretical perspective; further, this needs to be a theoretical perspective appropriate for understanding nursing phenomena.
3. **Review of literature** – should be logically organised and should include a discussion of the major variables. Importantly, Ryan-Wenger purports that the review of the literature needs to be more than a list of previous research findings; it is a critical review of the extant literature. Interestingly, the author warns of criticising the extant literature that may be used to support the findings of the new study.

4. **Research questions/hypothesis** – should be stated explicitly and not left to the reader to infer.
5. **Sample** – the target population must be described in order for the reader to determine how representative the sample is and thus how generalisable the findings are.
6. **Human or animal subject concerns** – the credibility of the research is enhanced if the researcher shows how the rights of the subjects were protected (i.e. the standard human rights protected in Codes of Ethics).
7. **Procedure** – should be described in a clear and precise way and should show how threats to internal and external validity were controlled.
8. **Operational definitions** – all nouns in the research questions/hypothesis should be operationally defined. The paper should also contain convincing information regarding the reliability and validity of the psychosocial/biomedical methods to measure the variables.
9. **Analysis** – needs to be enhanced by stating the alpha level (i.e. the level of significance) in advance of any analysis or interpretation of the results.
10. **Results** – should be addressed in order (as according to Ryan-Wenger, this adds to logical consistency). Also there should be enough information provided to evaluate the author's interpretation of the results.
11. **Interpretation** – the congruence between the findings in the study and the selected theoretical framework should be discussed.
12. **Potential for replication** – unfortunately, there do not appear to be any guidelines offered as to how the reviewer can evaluate the potential for replication.

Having described the key elements of Ryan-Wenger's approach, we next offer an example of the product of this approach and we then highlight some of the strengths and limitations of this approach.

Example 7

The paper reviewed was Verbosky-Cadena, S. V. (2006) Living among strangers: the needs and functioning of persons with schizophrenia residing in an assisted living facility. *Issues in Mental Health Nursing*, **27**, 25–42.

Abstract/overview

This paper reports on a study which wanted to describe the quality of care for people diagnosed with severe and persistent schizophrenia who reside in an assisted living facility. More specifically, in addition to the characteristics of this population, the paper intended to determine whether or not there was a relationship between resident characteristics and level of functioning, and the resultant needs of the residents. The study used a correlational, quasi-experimental design, sampled 58 residents and 16 care givers, and collected data using a combination of interviews, scales and instruments. The findings suggest that a typical profile of a resident is a 43-year-old, never-married Caucasian male, who never completed high school and who has had a history of severe mental health 'illness' for 21 years. Significant relationships were found between level of functioning and positive/negative symptoms, and medication knowledge.

Credibility of research report

1. **Writing style** – the article is written in a reasonable academic style. The sequence of sections is logically organized. The paper contains, however, a number of unanswered rhetorical questions which tend to detract from the overall quality of the writing style.
2. **Authors** – The paper does not include any information about the author which allows the degree of congruence between the clinical focus/area of study to be determined. The author appears to have completed her PhD in 1999, though there is no evidence of a track record of publications in the substantive area.
3. **Title of the research report** – according to the criteria identified by Ryan-Wenger, the title of the paper can be regarded as missing some key terms and also containing terms that detract from the credibility. The title does not include terms which identify the specific study design; the major variables are identified, as is the target population.
4. **Abstract** – the abstract does appear to include the research problem and the specific objectives of the study. The sample and major variables are also identified. No hypothesis is stated, and some detail of the method is also evident in the abstract. A summary of the results is built-in; however, the discussion of and implications arising from these results are not the strongest section of the abstract. Indeed, the relationship between the findings and the stated implications is tenuous at best and appears to require something of an 'intellectual leap' on the part of the reader.
5. **Problem** – the paper includes a section that identifies the research problem. However, it can be argued that there might be some conceptual slippage. The author refers to 'quality of care' and different levels of patient needs, yet the literature referred to to support this association actually refers to 'quality of life' – not quality of care. This is difficult to comprehend given that the theoretical framework used is Donabedian's (1982, 1988) work on quality of care, and there exists an additional substantial literature in the area of quality of care/psychiatric nursing that could have been drawn upon. Recent examples of this literature include Baradell (2001), Wright (2003) and Melvin *et al.* (2005).

Integrity of research method

1. **Logical consistency** – in terms of the congruence between the theoretical framework, review of literature, purpose, research questions, designs, operational definitions, analysis and interpretation of findings, certain sections appear

to share a firmer congruence than others. However, overall the degree of congruence between the separate sections of the study appears to be high. For example, the method/design chosen appears to be congruent with the stated research problem and hypotheses, and the instruments used appear to be congruent with the required information. On the other hand, in the review of the literature, the focus appears to be on the diagnosis and symptomology of schizophrenia, where such individuals reside, and the shift in where such people reside (from long-stay institutions to community). While this can be regarded as relevant background or contextual information, it says little or nothing about the existing work in the area and therefore might be regarded as lacking congruence with the rest of the study.

2. **Theoretical framework** – The theoretical framework of the research is Donabedian's (1982, 1988) work on 'Quality of Care' and it would be difficult to refute that there is a relationship between nursing and quality of care. Nevertheless, Donabedian's theoretical framework is not exclusive to nursing, and does not originate from any of the disciplines (fields of study) identified by Ryan-Wenger.

3. **Review of literature** – the review of literature did not appear to be the strongest section of the paper. As stated above, the literature review contained mainly contextual or background information; material which would perhaps have been better included as part of the justification for the study. The literature review did not include a list of previous research findings; neither then did it provide a critical review of the extant literature. Indeed, not one study was identified in the literature review which had attempted to examine quality of life or quality of care in people with schizophrenia, and recent examples of this literature are bounteous (e.g. Lehman, 1999; Ryan, 2004; Ware, 2004). For that matter, no studies that had attempted to measure quality of life and/or quality of care in other populations were included. This is a significant limitation of the study.

4. **Research questions or hypothesis** – The paper includes two research hypotheses (p. 29): 'a) there is a correlation among level of functioning, needs, symptoms of illness, medication knowledge and demographic variables; and b) the demographic and response variables are related to the level of functioning of participants with schizophrenia'. One can argue that this might have been expressed in a more clear, explicit form. For example, the reader is left wondering if the hypothesis refers to a positive or negative correlation (Peat, 2002; Hicks, 2004). It needs to be admitted that, according to Ryan-Wenger (1992), directional hypotheses are appropriate if there is sufficient theoretical and empirical support to predict the outcome, which perhaps accounts for the absence of directional hypotheses. However, given the absence of previous related studies cited in the literature review, and applying Ryan-Wenger's guidelines, which state that research questions are most appropriate when previous research findings are equivocal or if little is known about the topic, then it may have been more appropriate for the author to have couched the hypotheses as research questions.

5. **Sample** – information contained in the paper regarding the nature and composition of the target population appeared to be a little confusing. In the abstract, the author states that 58 ALF (Assisted Living Facility) residents with schizophrenia were sampled, *in addition to* [our emphasis] eight direct care givers. However, there is no further mention of the direct care-givers. The author (pp. 29/30) describes the sample as a stratified random sample, yet does not appear to indicate what the stratification refers to; presumably it refers to the number of different Assisted Living facilities from which the sample was drawn? There is also no indication of how the sample was randomised. To the credit of the author, the total number of residents living in Assisted Living Facilities is stated, and as there is no reference to any power calculations, the reader guesses/assumes that the figure of 58 (total sample) must have been the sample size predetermined to produce an alpha level of significance of >0.05. However, it would have enhanced the credibility of the study if this had been made explicitly clear. The sample appears to be representative and thus generalisable results are possible.

6. **Human or animal subject concerns** – the credibility of the author's research can be considered to be enhanced by the inclusion of material that refers directly to how the rights of the subjects were protected (Beauchamp and Childress, 2001).

7. **Procedure** – the reader felt that certain sections of the study's procedure could have been made clearer. For example, several of the procedures appear to be described in the 'Results' section and not the 'Procedures' section; it was not clear from the article if the measurements were taken only once (and thus cross-sectional; Polit et al., 2001) or more longitudinal. There did not appear to be any reference to threats to internal or external validity, which, given that this was a quasi-experimental design, is something of an oversight (Polit et al., 2001; Peat, 2002).

8. **Operational definitions** – the material to be considered which is subsumed under this subheading was mixed. Some of the operational definitions were either defined or described (schizophrenia, resident of an ALF), and yet some others did not appear to be – 'needs' and 'functioning' for example. It was somewhat confusing as to the nature of the 'intervention'; a phenomenon that would need to be part of the study in order for it to be correctly titled as a quasi-experimental design (Peat, 2002; Hicks, 2004). It was also unclear as to which variable constituted the independent variable. The paper did contain information regarding the psychosocial/biomedical instruments to measure the variables, though data pertaining to reliability and validity of the instruments was unclear/missing.

9. **Analysis** – as stated previously, the article did not appear to state the alpha level (i.e. the level of significance) in advance of any analysis or interpretation of the results. However, inspection of the results section (pp. 34–5) shows that there are several references to 'at the 0.05 significance level'. Therefore one might deduce that this was the *a priori* required level of significance (and indeed a significance level that is commonly used; Polit et al., 2001).

10. **Results** – the research hypotheses were indeed addressed in order. However, the explanation of the results sections was rather hard to follow. Here is an example: 'Variables that significantly explained the resident's level of functioning in the study were: present GAF ($F = 7.17, p = 0.01$), GAF within the past year ($F = 7.32, p = 0.009$)'. As a result, the reader was left wondering – has there been more than one measurement over a 'time-line?' This was further confused given that table five (level of function scores for the participants) did not indicate different time-line measurements.

11. **Interpretation** – this section of the paper, according to Ryan-Wenger's guidelines, was not the strongest section. The incongruence between the findings in the study and the selected theoretical framework was not discussed, but there again, this apparent incongruence had not been identified earlier in the paper either; therefore perhaps this was not regarded as incongruent for the author? The author appears to have undertaken a comparison of her findings with existing literature, a process regarded as essential by Ryan-Wenger, though this comparison revealed that, 'resident needs are not correlated with variable in this study. This finding is unlike what is reported in the literature' (p. 36). However, only one other study is cited. Given that additional literature does indeed exist in this substantive area, this perhaps casts doubt on any conclusions arising from comparing the findings with the extant literature. Further, it does appear that rather than engage in a searching discussion about why the findings were polarised with respect to the findings in the extant literature, the author instead focuses on exhorting formal mental health services to produce state-wide programs that address the needs identified in her study. Such 'grand' claims arising out of the findings of one study might be regarded as epistemologically premature (Popper, 1965; McKenna, 1997). When the author proceeds to discuss levels of functioning, there is more evidence of comparison with the extant literature and consistency in the findings (e.g. the relationship between duration of a person's 'illness' and lower levels of functioning). There was no evidence of 'paradigm effect' (Ryan-Wenger, 1992) in the paper, and this can be regarded as a strength. A further limitation of this section is that of the absence of any 'Limitations of the Study' section, which Ryan-Wenger asserts should be woven into the discussion of the findings.

12. **Potential for replication** – in the view of the reader, it would be possible to reproduce or replicate this study in a similar population, though it might not be possible to do so based only on the information that is provided in the paper; it is possible that the researcher would need to access the author's dissertation, where a more complete description of the study is likely to exist. However, the reader cannot help but wonder about and subsequently ask the 'So what?' question? Given that many of the findings described in this paper are concerned with the particular characteristics of a sample of people who live in ALFs, the reader is not sure of the international value of such findings. Furthermore, there may or may not be correlations between level of functioning and duration of 'illness' (or a range of other variables), but once again one is left wondering 'So what?'. Would it not be more appropriate to look at a range of

interventions and programs that go about meeting those needs (and subsequently evaluating the programs)? However, additional research that shows that the needs of many people living in ALFs are not being met is worthwhile, and that is to the credit of the author.

References

Baradell, J. G. (2001) Outcomes and satisfaction of patients of psychiatric clinical nurse specialists. *Journal of the American Psychiatric Nurses Association*, **7**(3), 77–85.

Beauchamp, T. L. and Childress, J. F. (2001) *Principles of Biomedical Ethics*, 5th edn. Oxford University Press, Oxford.

Donabedian, R. (1982) *Explorations in Quality Assessment and Monitoring: the Criteria and Standards of Quality (2)*, Health Administration Press, Ann Arbor, MI.

Donabedian, R. (1988) *Explorations in Quality Assessment and Monitoring: the Definition of Quality and Approaches to its Management*. Health Administration Press, Ann Arbor, MI.

Hicks, C. (2004) *Research Methods for Clinical Therapists: Applied Project Design and Appraisal*, 4th edn. Churchill Livingstone, Edinburgh.

Lehman, A. F. (1999) Quality of care in mental health: the case of schizophrenia: new therapies show great promise in treating persons with schizophrenia. The challenge is to get the treatment to the patient. *Health Affairs*, **18** (5), 52–65.

McKenna, H. P. (1997) *Nursing Theories and Models* Routledge, London.

Melvin, M., Hall, P. and Bienek, E. (2005) Practice development. Redesigning acute mental health services: an audit into the quality of inpatient care before and after service redesign in Grampian. *Journal of Psychiatric and Mental Health Nursing*, **12**(6), 733–8.

Peat, J. (2002) *Health Science Research: a Handbook of Quantitative Methods*. Sage, London.

Polit, D. P., Beck, C. T. and Hungler, B. P. (2001) *Essentials of Nursing Research: Methods, Appraisal and Utilization*, 5th edn. Lippincott, Philadelphia.

Popper, K. (1965) *Conjectures and Refutations: the Growth of Scientific Knowledge*. Harper & Row, New York.

Ryan, T. (2004) Long term care for serious mental illness outside the NHS: a study of out of area placements. *Journal of Mental Health*, **13**(4), 425–9.

Ware, N. C. (2004), Practitioner relationships and quality of care for low-income persons with serious mental illness. *Psychiatric Services*, **55**(5), 555–9.

Wright, E. R. (2003) The effect of organizational climate on the clinical care of patients with mental health problems. *Journal of Emergency Nursing*, **4**, 314–21.

Strengths and limitations of Ryan-Wenger's (1992) guidelines for critique of a research report

Strengths

■ The approach makes a very good point regarding the importance of missing information, stating that the *absence* (original emphasis) of variables affects the quality of the research.

- The suggestion of several reads of the paper, with a different focus for each read, is an interesting and infrequently encountered suggestion.
- The detail in what to look for, and how to determine the credibility of the 'Authors' section is also infrequently encountered and can be regarded as a strength.
- While the approach makes some rather 'concrete' statements, these (in the main) appear to be grounded in the cogent, theoretical, epistemological and philosophical literature.
- The detail in the 'Operational definitions' section, on which statistical tests to look for (according to the types of variable included in the study) is also infrequently encountered and can be regarded as a strength.
- It is possible that the author of the researcher paper reviewed may learn from a critique using Ryan-Wenger's approach, particularly if the author was attempting to adhere to the tenets of deductive approaches to research.
- Lastly in this section, while the approach is clearly only orientated towards evaluating quantitative studies, the author is completely open and 'up-front' about this, stating that this approach should not be applied to qualitative (inductive) studies. While clearly limiting the scope of this approach, this openness and honesty removes the chance of the approach being used inappropriately and we regard this as a strength.

Limitations

- As stated above, the approach makes comparisons against 'accepted standards', which begets questions about developments in methodology and method; accordingly a study that draws on a methodology and method outside of the normative methodological orthodoxy would then be evaluated as 'flawed' using Ryan-Wenger's approach.
- Insisting that some theoretical work is useful as a basis for nursing and other work is not, is a significant limitation; Ryan-Wenger's example does not include change management literature, social geography or business literature. One might purport that because nursing is inherently a 'human endeavour' any theoretical body of knowledge that speaks to or helps understand a human, or 'being' human or the world that humans live in, could also be useful.
- While the approach 'reluctantly' acknowledges that studies may be based on multi-theories, the stated preference is for 'a' (singular) theoretical framework. It is important to note that contemporary understandings of health related phenomena (e.g. consider the term biopsychosocial) invariably involve highly complex, multidimensional, multitheoretical models.

■ There are significant problems with an approach that advocates being 'careful' about criticising literature if it supports the findings of the current study, while at the same time advocating that literature that does not support the current study *should be* criticised.

Reference

Ryan-Wenger, N. M. (1992) Guidelines for critique of a research report. *Heart and Lung*, **21**(4), 394–401.

CHAPTER 7

Polit and Hungler's (1997) approach to critiquing nursing research

This chapter focuses on Polit and Hungler's (1997) approach to critiquing nursing research. It describes their guidelines (Box 7.1) and the five key areas that the reviewer needs to consider. To facilitate the application of this approach we have summarised the key issues in each of these areas into lists of questions. Following this we provide two detailed examples (drawing on the reviews carried out by the NPNR Journal Club). Having described the approach and provided examples, we then highlight some of the strengths and limitations of this approach.

Polit and Hungler (1997, p. 410) declare that a research critique is:
not just a review or summary of a study but rather a careful, critical appraisal of the strengths and limitations of a piece of research.

They argue that each research report has a number of important dimensions and that a thorough critique of the paper would include consideration of each of these dimensions. They describe these dimensions as: substantive and theoretical, methodologic, ethical, interpretive and presentational/stylistic. In addition to these five areas, Polit and Hungler (1997) provide a set of overall guidelines for critiquing research reports (Box 7.1) and guidelines for considering the interpretive dimensions of the study and the presentational dimensions of the study (Boxes 7.2 and 7.3).

Substantive and theoretical dimensions

1. Was the study important in terms of:
    A   The significance of the problem
    B   The soundness of the conceptualisations
    C   The appropriateness of the theoretical framework
    D   The creativity and insightfulness of the analysis

Box 7.1 Guidelines for the conduct of a written research critique (from Polit and Hungler, 1997)

1. Be sure to comment on the study's strengths as well as its limitations. The critique should be a balanced consideration of the worth of the research. Each research report has *some* [original emphasis] positive features. Be sure to find them and note them.
2. Give specific examples of the study's strengths and limitations. Avoid vague generalisations of praise and fault finding.
3. Try to justify your criticisms. Offer a rationale for how a different approach would have solved a problem that the researcher failed to address.
4. Be as objective as possible. Try to avoid being overly critical because you are not particularly interested in a topic or because you have a world view that is inconsistent with the underlying paradigm.
5. Be sensitive in handling negative comments. Try to put yourself in the shoes of the researcher receiving the critical appraisal. Do not be condescending or sarcastic.
6. Suggest realistic alternatives that the researcher (or future researchers) might want to consider. Don't just identify problems – offer some recommended solutions, making sure that the recommendations are practical ones.
7. Evaluate all aspects of the study – its substantive, theoretical, methodologic, ethical, interpretive and presentational dimensions.

---

2. Is the research problem relevant to nursing? Would it have been more appropriate for the study to have been conducted by a discipline other than nursing?

3. The researcher should ask: given what we know about this topic, is this research the right next step? (As knowledge development is often incremental and sequential, it is wise to avoid unnecessary repetition. However, the reviewer should consider: has the researcher taken several 'leaps ahead'?

4. Is the study question congruent with the methods used to address it?

5. Has the researcher appropriately placed the research problem into a larger theoretical context?

Methodologic dimensions

Four main design decisions in quantitative studies:

1. *Design*: Was the most appropriate design for the study used? Which design would provide the clearest and most meaningful results regarding the hypothesis/null hypothesis?
2. *Participants*: What was the composition of the sample? How large was the sample, was this adequate? How were they recruited, was this appropriate?
3. *Measures*: Which measuring instruments/tools were used? Consider: how can the variable under study be operationalised (isolated) and reliably/validly measured for each participant?
4. *Procedure*: How and when did the measurement(s) occur? What statistical analysis would provide the most test of the hypothesis?

Four main design questions in qualitative studies:

1. *Setting*: Where did the study take place and did this setting(s) enable the richest, deepest understanding of the phenomenon under study?
2. *Data*: What was (were) the source(s) of data? How was it gathered? Was this appropriate to the design or should other data options have been considered, both in terms of sources and methods of collection?
3. *Participants*: What was the composition of the sample? Were they selected according to sampling techniques congruent with qualitative approaches, i.e. purposeful, theoretical sampling? Did the choice of participants reflect the population who could provide a rich, deep thorough understanding of the phenomenon?
4. *Credibility*: Did the researcher make any efforts to establish the credibility or authenticity of his/her findings? How was this issue addressed?

Ethical dimensions

The key question within the ethical dimension is: was there any evidence within the research that the subject's human rights were violated in any way?

Polit and Hungler (1997) point out that there are two principal types of ethical transgression within research studies, and they describe these as inadvertent actions and purposeful (relatively) minor ethical violations.

Interpretive dimensions

Polit and Hungler (1997) describe a range of issues and questions which need to be considered in the interpretive dimension and summarise these with questions listed in Box 7.2.

Box 7.2 Guidelines for critiquing the interpretive dimensions of a research report (from Polit and Hungler 1997)

1. Does the discussion section offer conclusions or interpretations for all the important results?
2. Are the interpretations consistent with the results? Do the interpretations give due consideration to the limitations of the research methods?
3. What types of evidence in support of the interpretations does the researcher offer? Is that evidence persuasive? Are the results interpreted in light of findings from other studies?
4. Are alternative explanations for the findings mentioned, and is the rationale for their rejection presented?
5. In quantitative studies, does the interpretation distinguish between practical and statistical significance?
6. Are generalisations made that are not warranted on the basis of the sample used?
7. Does the researcher offer any implications of the research for nursing practice, nursing theory and/or nursing research? Are the implications appropriate, given the study's limitations?
8. Are specific recommendations for practice or future studies made? Are the recommendations consistent with the findings and consistent with the body of knowledge on the topic?

Presentational and stylistic dimensions

Polit and Hungler (1997) describe a range of issues and questions which need to be considered in the presentational and stylistic dimension and summarise these with questions listed in Box 7.3.

Box 7.3 Guidelines for critiquing the presentation of a research report (from Polit and Hungler, 1997)

1. Does the report include a sufficient amount of detail to permit a thorough critique of the study's purpose, conceptual framework, design and methods, handling of critical ethical issues, analysis of data and interpretation?
2. Is the report well written and grammatical? Are pretentious words or jargon used when a simpler wording would have been possible?
3. Is the report well organised, or is the presentation confusing? Is there an orderly presentation of ideas? Are transitions smooth, and is the report characterised by continuity of thought and expression?
4. Is the report sufficiently concise, or does the author include a lot of irrelevant detail? Are important details omitted?
5. Does the report suggest overt biases?
6. Is the report written using tentative language as befits the nature of the disciplined enquiry, or does the author talk about what the study did or did not prove?
7. Is sexist language avoided?
8. Does the title of the report adequately capture the key concepts of the population under investigation? Does the abstract (if any) adequately summarise the research problem, study methods, and important findings?

Example 8: The Network for Psychiatric Nursing Research Journal Club: Review from the 1st meeting.

The paper reviewed was Veeramah, V. (1995) A study to identify the attitudes and needs of qualified staff concerning the use of research findings in clinical practice within mental health care settings. *Journal of Advanced Nursing*, **22**, 855–61.

Abstract/overview

This paper reported on a small-scale exploratory survey which attempted to assess the attitudes and needs of qualified nurses working within mental health settings. A total of 150 questionnaires were sent to trained nurses working in the south-east of England and 118 questionnaires were returned, which indicates a response rate of 78%. The researcher claimed that the main findings were that although the vast majority of nurses in the study have a positive attitude to research, very few actually make significant use of research findings to enhance their practice. The author then lists some of the variables that seem to contribute to this state of affairs and points out that most of the nurses said they would be involved in research activities if the time was provided for them to do so.

Substantive and theoretical dimension

1A The identified research problem certainly warrants investigation, in that it appears to be 'covering new ground' or at the very least investigating an area that appears to be distinctly under-researched. Therefore the study can be regarded as important.

1B It appears that the paper did contain concepts that lacked definition or perhaps suffered from a lack of clarity. This was particularly noticeable in the introduction and the literature review. Some of the members wondered even if the author fully understood what was meant by research, as there appeared to be a confusion between evidence-based practice and research-based practice (McKenna et al., 2000). It might have been useful to include some definitions of what constitutes 'research-based practice' and the author could have included some extra detail in order to 'demystify' research. Furthermore, the crucial issue that nursing research should inform practice, not dictate practice, was absent.

1C There is little evidence of a theoretical framework within the study.

1D The members felt that there were many opportunities in this paper where the researcher could have been more creative and insightful, and in a sense had not 'extended him/herself' fully. These are explored in the Interpretive dimension section in more detail.

2. The research problem is highly relevant to nursing and this can be viewed as one of the strengths of the paper. The emphasis on evidence-based practice has clearly increased over recent years and it is thus not surprising that new journals (e.g. *Evidence Based Nursing*), a growing body of literature (e.g. Muir Gray, 1997) and centres for disseminating research evidence (e.g. the International Cochrane Collaboration) have also emerged. Consequently, few (if any) credible health care professionals would deny that sound evidence should be an integral part of clinical decision making. Therefore, while recognising that research-based practice is but one of the four components of evidence-based practice (McKenna et al., 2000), it is still appropriate and indeed necessary to investigate issues involved in the use of research- (and evidence-) based practice.

3. Opinion was divided amongst the members as to whether or not this research was the right 'next step'. The author ends the literature section by listing seven propositions. It should be noted that the researcher points out that these propositions are based mainly on literature reviews and are not well supported empirically. Nevertheless, it is evident that the researcher includes questions in the questionnaire that appear to be in response to the issues highlighted by these seven propositions (but not all of them). Therefore, it could be argued that the researcher is trying to build upon existing knowledge.

However, several questions were raised by the journal club members: why did the author not construct a questionnaire to address each of the seven propositions? If the researcher acknowledges that several of the propositions are not based on empirical study, does that not indicate a direction for study that the researcher could follow? Does the absence of any empirically based theory in these areas indicate the need for a qualitative study?

4. This was another question where opinion was mixed. It would appear to be entirely appropriate, having once decided that the study question is concerned with determining the 'research needs' of qualified staff, that a survey design is used to measure the extent and nature of these needs (Parahoo, 1997; Polit et al., 2001; Hicks, 2004). However, the researcher did not limit himself/herself to measuring the needs, and indeed the principal objective of the study was to assess the attitudes of the staff towards nursing research. Consequently, there may have been merit in exploring the different ways that attitudes may be measured and it was perhaps remiss of the researcher not to mention the significant difficulty and wide debate that surround the practice of measuring attitudes. This is explored in more detail in the Methodological dimensions section.

5. The researcher appears to have located the research problem within a larger theoretical context; namely the need for nursing to move towards being an evidence- (research-) based discipline.

Methodological dimension

Since the study purports to be using a quantitative method, the key questions relating to design, sample, measures and procedures are considered in this section.

1. The study uses a simple survey design, and whilst surveys have been used previously to investigate this phenomenon (Hunt, 1981; Lacey, 1994), it may not have been the most appropriate method. Attempts to measure attitudes present a range of methodological difficulties (Parahoo, 1997; Hicks, 2004), and it was felt by some members of the Journal Club that the paper might have benefited from some attention to this matter. The members' difficulty resides not in the ultimate choice of a survey, but rather the absence of any consideration of methodological options or consideration of the methodological difficulties in attempting to measure attitudes. It may have been worthwhile for the author to have explored alternative scoring systems, for example using questions with visual analogue scales or semantic differential scales, which have particular value in measuring subjective experiences, and this would have been more in keeping with measuring attitudes (Parahoo, 1997).

Alternatively, perhaps the use of focus groups could have been considered, since according to Roberts (1999), focus groups as a means of gathering (qualitative) data offers several advantages, particularly when trying to understand the behaviour, attitudes and perception of a group. These advantages include synergism, stimulation from other group members, security and speed. Additionally, the semi-structured nature of focus groups would have allowed the researchers to:

(a) let the focus group participants respond to one another as they discuss their attitudes towards research (and thus add to the richness and depth of the data) and (b) pick up on and subsequently follow any key issues or particular themes that emerged during the focus group.

A second alternative method that was suggested by the members was to use a triangulated design and combine the qualitative component with a subsequent quantitative survey. Using this design, the researcher would perhaps have first induced a theory of P/MH nurses' attitudes to research, and could then have measured the extent to which this theory was accurate for a wider population of P/MH nurses.

2. It is difficult to comment on the composition of the sample, as the precise details of the sample are not included in the paper. This can be regarded as an over-sight and limitation of the paper. The researcher stated that he/she attempted to sample as many qualified P/MH nurses from specific clinical areas (both in-patient and community areas) as possible. Unfortunately, the paper contains no breakdown of how many questionnaires were distributed to each clinical area, or a breakdown of community/hospital distribution. Consequently, members were left guessing how the questionnaires were distributed, and indeed who they were distributed to.

3. It appeared that the author had largely attempted to replicate the design used by Leach (1994) (cited in the reviewed paper) and had augmented this question-naire with two further questions. Members stated that the additional questions added something extra to the original questionnaire, but felt that the tool could have withstood further refinement. For example:

- had the tool undergone any tests for validity?
- were the terms used in the questionnaire operationally defined?
- some of the questions appear to have an element of ambiguity and thus may cause confusion. In Question 1 for example, are the respondents being asked to agree/disagree with the 'research-based' aspect, the 'profession' aspect or both? In Question 2, what does, 'research activity' refer to? Conducting re-search, implementing research or reading research?

4. There is no mention in the paper of when the measurements occurred and the members were left assuming that the results refer to a 'single time point' meas-urement.

Ethical dimensions

The researcher does state that the necessary permissions were gained from all the appropriate managers; however, there appears to be no mention of ethical considerations. Given that the research appeared to take place (at least in part) on NHS premises, and given the Department of Health's (1991) guidelines on research and Local Research Ethics Committees (LRECs), it would have been prudent for the researcher to submit the research proposal to the LREC for approval.

Interpretive dimension

1. The view of the members was that the discussion section did not offer conclusions or interpretations of all the important results. The discussion appeared to be largely a reiteration of the findings and some comparison of the results to the studies cited in the literature review. Suggestions regarding what the researcher might have included in the discussion are listed in Question 7.
2. The limited interpretations appear to be congruent with the results and are considered within the context of the limitations.
3. The researcher draws upon the evidence of the previous findings of the studies cited in the literature review.
4. It does not appear that alternative explanations are offered. One such alternative explanation might have been an argument that suggested that those nurses who feel more positive towards research are more likely to complete and return a questionnaire of this nature. Indeed, perhaps the absence of such consideration may even cast doubt on the validity of the findings, and this led members to wonder whether the most appropriate question had been asked. Some members felt that a more appropriate question to ask was; 'What do nurses understand by the term research?'. Perhaps an important question that the researcher could have asked of the data was: 'How easy would it have been for nurses to say they have a negative attitude towards research?', particularly when nurses are frequently told, in policy documents, published papers and in their pre- and post-registration education, that research is 'good' and should be embraced.
5. There does not appear to be any mention of statistical significance, but the researcher did state that he/she intended to avoid 'jargon' and keep the analysis simple in order that the majority of nurses might understand it.
6. There does not appear to be any evidence of unwarranted generalisations within the discussion.
7. There is evidence of only limited discussion of the implications for nursing practice/theory/research. Members highlighted that there are so many relevant issues relating to this matter and the findings of the research, and felt that the researcher rather 'sold himself/herself short.' For example, the researcher could have considered: is research-based practice always something to strive for (McKenna et al., 2000) and if not, how might this consideration have affected the results? Is there the body of research in P/MH nursing for the nurses to be using in their practice? (Ward et al., 2000) Has the most valuable/useful or most appropriate type of knowledge been uncovered in the research that has

been conducted for nursing, and if not, how might this affect the nurses' attitudes towards and utilisation research findings? Several authors have alluded to the different types of knowledge that nurses need (see Benner, 1984; Pearson, 1992; McKenna, 1997; Polit et al., 2001) and if nursing research is producing knowledge that has only limited relevance or application to clinical practice, then this may have an impact on the nurses' attitudes towards those research findings (Cutcliffe, 1998). There is another question that warrants consideration, and that is: would it always be in the best interests of nurses to be aware of the latest research findings? That is, would the nurses be placed in a dichotomous position if the research evidence indicated one way of practice and the organisation or medical colleagues advocate another? A crucial issue which the members felt was a particularly significant omission was that research should inform practice – not dictate it (McKenna et al., 2000).

8. The paper does make specific recommendations, and these were felt to have sense and value. However, while they appear to have some resonance with the results, they do not appear to have been uncovered through the research process. That is, many of the recommendations do not appear to have evolved directly from the results, and consequently the members felt that some of these had an element of impracticability.

Presentational and stylistic dimension

1. The report contains most of the detail required, but some important details appear to be missing. For example: the paper contains no (null) hypothesis or research question (however, it does contain a series of study objectives), there is a distinct absence of detailed consideration of any ethical issues, and members felt that a thorough discussion of the implications of the results was absent.

2. Members described the paper as reasonably well written and noted that it appears to have been written purposefully to enable the reader's understanding. (Indeed, the author makes such claims within the paper.) Consequently, one of the strengths of the paper can be considered to be the absence of unnecessary jargon or tautology. However, in attempting to be, as the researcher states, 'as simple as possible' (p. 858), the paper perhaps loses rigour.

3. In the main the paper had a logical flow and conformed to the standard format of introduction, literature review, methods, results, discussion, conclusion (Tierney, 1991; Polit et al., 2001). However, as stated above, the collection of recommendations at the end of the paper appear to be based on a review of the literature, and not necessarily on the findings. Therefore the inclusion of these recommendations at this point in the paper might be regarded as inappropriate.

4. Members described the paper as being reasonably well organised and there was no evidence of irrelevant detail. The author acknowledges the omission

of an important detail: the total number of the sample. The lack of information concerning the distribution of the questionnaire was thought to be an oversight. The paper left the members assuming that each participant only filled in one questionnaire each, yet this is not made clear in the paper, and importantly, this might be because the researcher could not be sure this was the case. Hence some more detail about the distribution and subsequent collection of the questionnaires may have helped.

5. The paper does not appear to contain any evidence of overt biases.
6. The researcher uses tentative language throughout the report, although it should be noted the members felt that, in places, the report had almost an apologetic feel with expressions such as; 'unfortunately, although the study was small scale... despite the sample size'.
7. The was no evidence of sexist language within the report.
8. The title and abstract both appear to be clear and concise.

References

Benner, P. (1984) *From Novice to Expert: Excellence and Power in Clinical Nursing*. Addison-Wesley, Menlo Park.

Cutcliffe, J. R. (1998) Is psychiatric nursing research barking up the wrong tree? *Nurse Education Today*, **18**, 257–8.

Department of Health (1991) *Local Research Ethics Committees*. Department of Health/HMSO, London.

Hicks, C. (2004) *Research Methods for Clinical Therapists: Applied Project Design and Analysis*, 4th edn. Churchill Livingstone, Edinburgh.

Hunt, J. (1981) Implications for nursing practice: the use of research findings. *Journal of Advanced Nursing*, **6**, 189–94.

Lacey, E. A. (1994) Research utilization in nursing practice – a pilot study. *Journal of Advanced Nursing*, **19**, 987–95.

McKenna, H. P. (1997) *Nursing Theories and Models*. Routledge, London.

McKenna, H. P., Cutcliffe, J. R. and McKenna, P. (2000) Evidence based practice: demolishing some myths. *Nursing Standard*, **14**(16), 39–42.

Muir Gray, J. A. (1997) *Evidence-Based Health Care*. Churchill Livingstone, Edinburgh.

Parahoo, K. (1997) *Nursing Research: Principles, Process and Issues*. Macmillan, London.

Pearson, A. (1992) Knowing nursing: emerging paradigms in nursing. In: *Knowledge for Nursing* (eds. K. Robinson and B Vaughan). Butterworth-Heinemann, Oxford.

Polit, D. P., Beck, C. T. and Hungler, B. P. (2001) *Essentials of Nursing Research: Methods, Appraisal and Utilization*, 5th edn. Lippincott, Philadelphia.

Roberts, P. (1999) Planning and running a focus group. *Nurse Researcher*, **4**, 78–82.

Tierney, A. J. (1991) Reporting and disseminating research. In: *The Research Process in Nursing*, 2nd edn (ed. D. Cormack), pp. 318–28. Blackwell Scientific, Oxford.

Ward, M., Cutcliffe, J. R. and Gournay, K. (2000) *The Nursing, Midwifery and Health Visiting Contribution to the Continuing Care of People with Mental Health Problems: a Review and UKCC Action Plan*. UKCC, London.

Example 9: The Network for Psychiatric Nursing Research Journal Club: Review from the 12th meeting

The paper reviewed was Whittington, R. and Wykes, T. (1994) An observational study of associations between nurses behaviour and violence in psychiatric hospitals. *Journal of Psychiatric and Mental Health Nursing*, 1, 85–92.

Abstract/overview

This paper described a cyclic model of violence to psychiatric nurses and then reports on a partial test of the model. The paper argued that stress induced by exposure to violence leads to impaired staff performance and adoption of behaviours which make the re-occurrence of violence more likely. The paper then reports how the researchers tested part of this model by proposing that certain staff behaviours (e.g. expressing verbal hostility) would be associated with an increased risk of assault. The paper then reports that there was some evidence of the proposed association and the researchers then claim that they discuss the implications of these findings for psychiatric nursing.

Substantive and theoretical dimension

1A The research area certainly warrants investigation. Violence continues to be a cause for concern within the National Health Service (NHS); indeed recent evidence indicates that the problem of violence towards nurses is increasing (Health Advisory Advisory Committee, 1987; Crichton, 1995; Department of Health, 2001). Consequently, any study that potentially contributes to a greater understanding of the dynamics and processes involved and thus helps to reduce the incidence of violence can be regarded as a significant study.

1B Opinion was divided on this matter. The paper posits an interesting model and few would doubt that the nurses' feelings and resulting behaviour could have an effect on client violence. However, the paper presents a rather simplistic model, and importantly omits many additional variables that could be similarly involved or contribute to the exacerbation of violence, e.g. experiential learning, clinical supervision (Cutcliffe, 1999), and cultural or organisational factors (Morrison, 1990).

1C Members again reported some concerns about the theoretical framework, given the concerns outlined in response to 1B. There was also the feeling that the model may contain an element of disciplinary prejudice. Examination of the approach to understanding and exploring that appears to be preferred within the discipline of psychology appears to emphasise the following process. Psychologists, in the main, look to individual behaviour to explain outcomes and decontextualise the material. Then they attempt to generalise to the wider population. Members wondered if this paper (given that one of the authors was a psychologist) might be one example of that process.

1 D Opinion was varied concerning the insightfulness and creativity of the analysis. Some members felt that the model represented an attempt to translate theories/ideas of stress and coping, into simplistic and unlikely scenarios in avoidant and confrontative coping. Other members felt that only limited empirical work has been undertaken which considers the possible effects of nurses' feelings and behaviours on client violence, and thus this paper maybe offers insight into such dynamics.

2. The research is clearly appropriate to nursing and one of the strengths of the paper was the researchers' willingness to address potentially awkward and yet highly relevant questions.

3. Opinion was divided with regard to this question. Some members felt that, given the relative lack of empirical work in this area, a qualitative method was indicated. Such a position is supported by the well-documented argument that a qualitative method is indicated when little or nothing is known about the phenomenon (see Dickoff and James, 1968; Munhall, 1993; Morse and Field, 1995; Polit et al., 2001). Other members felt that perhaps positing and subsequently testing simplistic hypotheses (i.e. there is a relationship between client violence, the nurse's feelings and the nurse's behaviour) was an appropriate choice. However, while it may have been appropriate to posit hypotheses, it should be noted that the members felt the model was too simplistic and failed to take account of the many confounding variables.

4. Given the question posed by the researchers, that certain types of nurse behaviour are more associated with violence by psychiatric clients than other types of behaviour, it was appropriate to use a quantitative, deductive method, in that the question is concerned with measurement and testing (Parahoo, 1997).

5. The researchers alluded to the larger theoretical context in terms of the ramifications of violence within the NHS, but only to a limited extent. However, they have attempted to locate the study, or at least link the study, to the wider formal area of 'stress and coping'.

Methodological dimension

Since the study purports to be using a quantitative method, the key questions relating to design, sample, measures and procedures are considered in this section.

1. The design was appropriate to the study question and provided some data that would enable the hypotheses to be tested. However, given the wide range of confounding variables and interactions of variables that could impact on client violence, it is debatable that the method used provided the clearest and most meaningful results. For example, there are arguments that posit violence as having a biological basis (Kreuz and Rose, 1972); that indicate the 'organisation's' role and culture in perpetuating violence (Morrison, 1990); and that use 'social learning' theories as the basis for explaining violence (Bandura, 1973). Given the possible interaction of these and other influences on client violence, the mem-

bers doubted that the design used in this study provided the clearest and most meaningful results.

Therefore, as an alternative, the researchers might have considered either a qualitative method or a different quantitative method. The choice of a qualitative method would have enabled the researchers to ask the clients: 'Tell me about your experiences of the nursing staff and if/how their behaviour contributes to client violent behaviour'. An alternative quantitative method would have involved the use of a survey and could have asked the clients to indicate from a range of nursing responses/behaviours the ones that would contribute to client violent behaviour.

2. The sample had two 'tiers' and consisted of certain wards and certain individuals on the wards. The nurses were selected by chance in that they happened to be on duty when the observations were made. However, the researchers state that the sample of nurses was representative of the overall population on the wards in terms of grade and sex.

With regard to the sample of wards, there are significant problems with designating wards as violent or non-violent, not least because of the ambiguity around defining an incident as violent (Cutcliffe, 1999; Turnbull, 1999). Indeed, the researchers made reference to this difficulty themselves. However, in the absence of any previous empirical work on which to base sampling decisions (i.e. previous studies could have determined that certain wards could be designated as violent and non-violent as a result of the wards meeting certain evidence-based criteria), the researchers have made some attempt to differentiate between such wards. Perhaps it would have been prudent for the researchers to acknowledge the limitations of their attempts to differentiate between violent and non-violent wards. Other members wondered, given the hypothesis and the bulk of the results, why such differentiations had been made at all.

3. The detail provided by the authors concerning the measures used was thought to be a strength of the paper. One minor point was raised with regard to the 'availability' measure. It was pointed out that nurses could well be unavailable to clients because they were engaged in therapeutic activity and thus not necessarily distancing themselves as a result of the stress they were feeling (as the researchers allude to).

4. The procedure used for measurement was also thought to be a strength of the paper, although the reviewed paper made no reference to the Hawthorne effect (Polit and Hungler, 1997; Hicks, 2004; Peat, 2002) and this was thought to be an oversight.

Ethical dimension

The paper contains no mention of consideration of ethical issues or ethical approval. This was felt to be a major limitation of the paper. For examples, members wondered about how the researcher might have responded if he had witnessed any purposeful provocation of a client (McHale and Gallagher, 2003).

Interpretive dimension

1. and 2. Members stated that the discussion contained some interpretation of what appear to be important results, yet it also contained some contradictions. For example, the researchers suggest that charge nurses were the least 'available' grade of nurse, yet tended to speak to clients more and were also at high risk of assault. On the other hand, enrolled nurses were a highly 'available' grade of nurse, made more rejecting statements, and used touch more often, yet were less at risk of assault. Perhaps what this discussion could have mentioned, given the confounding and often conflicting relationships between variables, is that simplistic proposed causal relationships do not offer a complete understanding of the processes, dynamics and interactions involved in violence between clients and staff.

3. The researchers draw upon previous empirical work in this substantive area. However, it may be worth noting that of the six references used in the discussion, four of the papers referenced were written by the author(s) of the current paper.

4. The researchers make reference to some of the contradictions in their findings, but then, instead of positing these as evidence to reject their model and hypotheses (and thus consider alternative explanations) they attempt to justify why these findings may have occurred and this results in much unsupported casual hypothesising.

5. The study includes 'P' values and distinguishes between practical and statistical significance (Peat, 2002; Hicks, 2004).

6. The study does not make any unwarranted generalisations.

7. Members felt that the paper contained important implications for psychiatric/ mental health nursing practice, yet these were largely implicit in the paper. Only the final paragraph of the discussion section contained any explicit indication of the implications and thus further attention to the implications may have been advisable. If, as the researchers posit, there appear to be some staff who use certain behaviours which provoke (or contribute to) client violence, then this has clear education and training implications. For example, self awareness or awareness raising is often regarded as an integral component of P/MH nurse preparation (Burnard, 1999; Barker, 2003) and many approaches exist to facilitate an increase in awareness (Heron, 1990; Duck, 1992). It is possible that the nurses who engage in behaviour that provokes client violence may do so unknowingly. (Indeed, if such behaviour is engaged in knowingly, then that raises a whole series of additional training/education issues!) However, if one accepts that the nurses are acting unknowingly, then the need for further self-awareness training becomes very clear. Furthermore, while there is little consensus in the literature on the practice of de-escalation (Patterson et al., 1997), few authors in this substantive area would disagree that an awareness of the nurse's feelings and resultant behaviour is inextricably linked to the practice of de-escalation.

The argument goes like this: if nurses are unaware of their own behaviour (e.g. use of touch, eye contact, body posture, verbal behaviours), then how can they engage competently in de-escalation techniques, since much of this practice involves monitoring oneself and adjusting potentially provocative actions?

Additionally, if we accept the researchers' argument that nurses who feel stressed may be more likely to engage in distancing behaviours and thus inadvertently provoke further violent actions, then there is a clear indication that nurses require support systems and methods of dealing with stress. The need for formal support systems for nurses who deal with violent incidents has been highlighted many times in the literature. Arguments proposing the introduction of post-incident counselling or de-briefing services (Ryan and Poster, 1993; Turnbull, 1993; Wykes & Mezey, 1994; Thomas, 1995) and the continuing need for clinical supervision (Cutcliffe, 1999) are perhaps the most common, and therefore it might have benefited the reviewed paper if further attention had been given to these particular service/education implications.

8. The paper contains limited recommendations for practice and for further study, stating only that further research is required to evaluate the importance of interpersonal behaviours in this significant problem. Additional implications that perhaps warranted discussion have been outlined in response to Question 7. Supplementary areas or issues for further study that the authors could have considered include: research aimed at understanding how nurses feel following client violence; how they deal with any resultant stress; how any residual stress affects their subsequent interactions; how clients feel when they perceive nurses behaving in avoidant or provocative ways; how the culture of the ward/unit may contribute to violence; and how prepared or trained nurses feel in engaging with potentially violent clients.

Presentational dimension

1. Members felt that, on the whole, the paper contains enough information to allow a thorough critique of the study's purpose, conceptual framework, design, methods, analysis and interpretations. However, there was a distinct absence of information regarding ethical issues and ethical considerations.
2. The report was written in a good academic style.
3. The report is, in the main, well organised and has a logical structure. The addition of a clearer conclusion section was suggested by some members.
4. The report is concise and does not include irrelevant detail.
5. Members felt that the paper did appear to contain some evidence of overt bias, and that was a bias towards the validity and accuracy of the proposed model. Evidence of this bias was in the form of the researcher's apparent unwillingness to consider alternative explanations or to consider using the evidence obtained as the basis for rejecting their model, and their apparent attempts to justify why these anomalous findings might have occurred.

6. The report uses tentative language as befitting of the nature of disciplined enquiry.
7. Sexist language is avoided.
8. Members felt the title was an accurate reflection of the content of the paper. The abstract however, did not appear to provide a description of the methods employed.

References

Bandura, A. (1973) *Aggression: a Social Learning Analysis*. Prentice Hall, New Jersey.

Barker, P. (2003) Person-centred care: the need for diversity In: *Psychiatric and Mental Health Nursing: the Craft of Care* (ed. P. Barker), pp. 3–9. Arnold, London.

Burnard, P. (1999) *Counselling Skills for Healthcare Professionals*, 3rd edn. Chapman & Hall, London.

Crichton, J. (1995) A review of psychiatric inpatient violence. In: *Psychiatric Patient Violence: Risk and Response* (ed. J. Crichton). Duckworth, London.

Cutcliffe, J. R. (1999) Qualified nurses' lived experiences of violence perpetrated by individuals suffering from enduring mental health problems: a hermeneutic study. *International Journal of Nursing Studies*, **36**, 105–16.

Department of Health (2001)

Dickoff, J. and James, P. (1968) A theory of theories: a position paper. *Nursing Research*. **17**(3), 197–203.

Duck, S. (1992) *Human Relationships*, 2nd edn. Sage, London.

Health Services Advisory Committee (1987) *Violence to staff in the Health Service*. HMSO, London.

Heron, J. (1990) *Helping the Client: a Creative Practical Guide*. Sage, London.

Hicks, C. (2004) *Research Methods for Clinical Therapists: Applied Project Design and Analysis*, 4th edn. Churchill Livingstone, Edinburgh.

Kreuz, L. E. and Rose, R. M. (1972) Assessment of aggressive behaviour and plasma testosterone in a young population. *Psychometric Medicine*. **34**, 321–2.

McHale, J. and Gallagher, A. (2003) *Nursing and Human Rights*. Butterworth-Heinemann, Edinburgh.

Morrison, E. F. (1990) The tradition of toughness: a study of non-professional nursing care in psychiatric nursing settings. *Image: Journal of Nursing Scholarship*, **22**(1), 32–8.

Munhall, P. L. (1993) Language and nursing research. In: *Nursing Research: a Qualitative Perspective* (eds. P. L. Munhall and C. O. Boyd). National League for Nursing Press, New York.

Morse, J. M. and Field, P. A. (1995) *Qualitative Research Methods for Health Professionals*, 2nd edn. Sage, London.

Patterson, B., Leadbetter, D. and McComish, A. (1997) De-escalation in the management of aggression and violence. *Nursing Times*, **93**(36), 58–61.

Peat, J. (2002) *Health Science Research: a Handbook of Quantitative Methods*. Sage, London.

Polit, D. P., Beck, C. T. and Hungler, B. P. (2001) *Essentials of Nursing Research: Methods, Appraisal and Utilization*, 5th edn. Lippincott, Philadelphia.

Ryan, J. and Poster, E. (1993) Workplace violence. *Nursing Times*, **89**(48), 38–41.

Thomas, B. (1995) Risky business. *Nursing Times*, **91**(7), 52–4.

Turnbull, J. (1993) Victim support. *Nursing Times*, **89**(23), 30–2.

Turnbull, J. (1999) Violence to staff: Who is at risk? In: *Aggression and Violence: Approaches to Effective Management* (eds. J. Turnbull and B. Patterson). Macmillan, London.

Wykes, T. and Mezey, G. (1994) Counselling for victims of violence. In: *Violence and Healthcare Professionals* (ed. T. Wykes), pp. 180–98. Chapman & Hall London.

Strengths and limitations of Polit and Hungler's approach

Strengths

- This is a very thorough and comprehensive approach. Furthermore, as this is the most recent of the four approaches we included (in the first edition), it perhaps indicates the evolutionary or developmental nature of approaches to critiquing research, wherein this approach has built upon the earlier approaches and has managed to address some of the limitations of these.
- The dimensions that have the detailed guidelines are thorough.
- It appears to give consideration to most of the fundamental components that each research report should make reference to.
- The approach does not have a 'sequential' 'step by step' method that could mirror the reading of the article. For example, questions asked of the title and abstract occur at the very end of the guidelines. Consequently, the reviewer is likely to need to read all the paper before any comment can be made and this may necessitate re-reading several sections. This may add to the rigour of the critique (while others may regard this as a limitation.)
- It does contain some research terminology, but this is not excessive or inappropriate. However, this does necessitate the reviewer having some understanding of basic concepts and practices within research.
- If a reviewer follows and subsequently addresses each of the questions contained within each of the five dimensions, then it is very likely that the author of the research paper reviewed may learn from a critique using Polit and Hungler's approach.
- As with Morrison's approach, Polit and Hungler's approach encourages the reviewer(s) to think about how the findings in the reviewed paper(s) may impact on nursing practice.
- The approach includes many useful and thought-provoking questions within the headings.
- The approach allows room for the data and/or argument to be introduced to support the reviewer's criticisms/observations and suggestions for improvement.

Limitations

- The approach provides lists of questions/guidelines for the interpretive and presentational dimensions, and yet does not provide lists/guidelines for the other three dimensions. It does not explain why this is the case. This leaves reviewers wondering whether Polit and Hungler are suggesting a greater 'weighting' for these dimensions? They do not appear to make this case explicitly.

■ As with the other approaches, this appears to be quantitatively orientated, in that the reviewer is encouraged to ask specific questions of quantitative studies e.g. in quantitative studies, does the interpretation distinguish between practical and statistical significance? And, are generalisations made that are not warranted on the basis of the sample used? However, the reviewer is not encouraged to ask questions specific to qualitative studies. However, unlike the three previous approaches, this approach does ask specific (and separate) methodological questions for both qualitative and quantitative studies.

■ Some of the specific guidelines might be considered to be repetitive.

■ As Polit and Hungler themselves point out, a critique should highlight the positive elements of a study in addition to the limitations. However, the lists of questions in the guidelines appear to usher the reviewer into considering the limitations more than the strengths.

Reference

Polit, D. F. and Hungler, B. P. (1997) *Essentials of Nursing Research: Methods, Appraisal and Utilization*, 4th edn. Lippincott, Philadelphia.

CHAPTER 8

Polit, Beck and Hungler's (2001) approach to critiquing qualitative nursing research

This chapter focuses on Polit *et al.*'s (2001) approach to critiquing qualitative nursing research. Given that this 2001 work is a development of the earlier Polit and Hungler texts on nursing research, it is not surprising that this text builds upon the guidelines provided in earlier versions (see Chapter 7) and reiterates the need to examine five key areas that the reviewer needs to consider. In addition to these, Polit *et al.*'s revised work reflects the trends described in Chapter 1, namely that of the nursing academe appearing to embrace methodological pluralism and that of the growing recognition of the value of qualitative studies. Accordingly, Polit *et al.*'s work includes an additional section that refers to the processes of interpreting qualitative results (or results/findings obtained) from qualitative research studies and it describes how these interpretations are woven into a critique.

Interestingly, Polit *et al.* (2001) purport that it is difficult for a reviewer to interpret qualitative findings thoroughly as a result of the researcher being selective about the amounts and types of data included in the report; nevertheless, they advocate that the reviewer should still attempt to ascertain the credibility of the findings. In so doing, Polit *et al.* (2001, p. 412) adopt a somewhat methodologically problematic (some qualitative research experts have argued 'out of date') approach to establishing the credibility of qualitative findings and urge the reviewer to examine the paper for evidence of:

peer debriefings, member checks, audits and triangulation.

Polit *et al.* (2001, p. 412) do offer a most useful suggestion when they state:

In thinking about the believability of qualitative results, as with quantitative results, it is advisable to adopt the posture of a person who needs to be persuaded and to expect the researcher to marshal solid evidence with which to persuade you.

The additional sections that Polit *et al.* (2001) describe for critiquing qualitative research findings are: the meaning of qualitative results, the importance of qualitative results, the transferability of qualitative results and the implications of qualitative results.

The meaning of qualitative results

According to Polit *et al.* (2001) efforts should be made to 'validate' the qualitative analysis, as this will in turn help 'validate' the findings, given that the meaning of the data flows from the process of data analysis. As a result, Polit *et al.* imply that examination of how the data have been analysed and similarly, the congruence between the particular method(s) of data analysis and resultant induced findings, can speak to the credibility of the findings.

The importance of qualitative results

As with any particular research question or research study, Polit *et al.* (2001) assert that the phenomenon investigated must be worthy of study: it must be of enough interest to warrant scrutiny. The often cited argument epistemological argument that 'little is known about the phenomenon' may not be sufficient grounds on its own. Polit *et al.* (2001) also predicate that the reviewer also needs to give attention to whether or not the findings themselves are trivial, suggesting that the reviewer might gauge the findings according to whether they are adding something new to the extant knowledge base. A further issue that should be looked at is the naming of labels, themes and/or categories. Polit *et al.* (2001) encourage reviewers to ask themselves whether these names represent an insightful construct; something that transcends what they term 'common knowledge.[1]

The transferability of qualitative results

Polit *et al.* (2001) declare that even though qualitative researchers do not attempt to produce generalisable findings, the reviewer should still consider the applica-

---

1 The authors of this book were surprised that the issue of parsimony was not included. Namely – the question of whether or not the findings/theory have been described/expressed in the smallest number of theoretical pieces, thus aiding understanding; more literally in science, parsimony is a preference for the least complex explanation for an observation.

tion of the findings to other contexts and settings; otherwise, Polit *et al.* argue, the findings have no usefulness.[2] The reviewer is urged to consider: what other types of settings and contexts would you expect to the phenomenon studied to be experienced and/or manifest? As a result, Polit *et al.* urge the reviewer to undertake an assessment of the detail provided regarding the context of the study in which the data were collected. If there is sufficient detail of the context in the original study, this will then enable a comparison to be made with other like contexts and thus speak to the transferability of the findings.

The implications of qualitative results

Polit *et al.* (2001) purport that if the reviewer believes the findings have met the conditions of the three previous sections, then the reviewer can go on to consider the implications. These implications, as with any other form or type of research finding, have several domains or dimensions of implication: further research, practice-related and theoretical implications. The reviewer is exhorted to consider whether or not the study could be expanded in a meaningful way? If the results are meaningful/important enough, does this merit the development of a formal measuring instrument or the need to test the emerging theory by means of a controlled quantitative study?[3]

Having described the key elements of Polit *et al.*'s approach, we next offer an example of the product of this approach. We then highlight some of the strengths and limitations of this approach.

Example 10

The paper reviewed was Rahm, G. B., Renck, B. and Ringsberg, K. C. (2006) 'Disgust, disgust beyond description' – shame cues to detect shame in disguise, in interviews with women who were sexually abused during childhood. *Journal of Psychiatric and Mental Health Nursing*, 13(1), 100–9.

---

2 Perhaps Polit *et al.* are referring to idiographic generalisability, but this is not made clear.

3 Here the authors of this book argue that Polit *et al.* have fallen into the often mistaken position of assuming that qualitative research exists *only* as a precursor to a quantitative study and cannot exist in and of itself as a valuable/useful addition to the literature.

Abstract/overview

This paper reports on a study which attempted to explore how women exposed to sexual abuse during childhood verbally express unacknowledged overt and covert shame. The study used a mainly qualitative method with semi-structured interviews, and ten women who attended a self-help group for sexual abuse agreed to participate and provide the data. The interview data were subsequently coded for incidences of shame by identifying code words and phrases. These words were sorted into six shame indicator groups and then categorised into aspects of shame, and the frequency of these words/phrases was also counted. Shame was found to be present and negatively influencing the lives of all the women. The authors conclude by stating that psychiatric services need to acknowledge both shame and sexual abuse in their clinical work in order to help them work through it.

Substantive and theoretical dimensions

1A There is little (if any) doubt within contemporary mental health care literature that problems arising from sexual abuse during childhood are not only common but also related to many serious mental health problems (see Hasse and Magnassun (2005) for a recent comprehensive review).

1B. The study includes a robust examination of the existing theoretical work and some of the empirical work; indeed, the extant literature related to shame appears to be fairly extensive and well established.

1C The study does not appear to be based on a theoretical framework.

1D Perhaps as result of recognising that there is a well-established body of work, it was felt that the study lacked creativity and insightfulness. Indeed, the relationship between having being a victim of sexual abuse and the resultant sense of shame seems rather obvious. Additionally, while the findings did have spontaneous validity (Kvale, 1996) for the reviewers, they did not appear to be adding much new information or adding much to our existing understanding.

2. The research problem is clearly relevant to P/MH nursing, and for that matter any discipline that is involved in providing mental health care, as a result, having a multidisciplinary mental health research team conduct the study appears to be a strength.

3. Given that we already appear to have a fairly solid knowledge base about the link between sexual abuse in childhood and a residual sense of shame, a further qualitative study such as this may not have been the most appropriate next step. Perhaps of greater utility would have been some work around how mental health practitioners might be able to help alleviate this sense of shame and/or the development of instruments that could accurately measure shame.

4. The study question is, at least in part, congruent with the methods used to address it; though if the researchers were adamant that they wished to undertake the study using a qualitative method (and that appears the case, given the comments on p. 108), it might have been more advantageous to use a 'pure'

qualitative method rather than the somewhat awkward methodological blend or hybrid that the authors have actually used.

5. As stated above, the researcher has linked the study with the existing theoretical and empirical work on shame, but does not base the study on an existing theoretical framework.

Methodologic dimension: four main design questions in qualitative studies

1. **Setting**: The research took place in Sweden and drew a purposeful sample from women who had contacted autonomous self-help groups for women with self-reported experiences of sexual abuse during childhood. Accordingly, the sample can be regarded as highly capable of providing a rich, deep insight into the experiences being investigated (Morse, 1998; Streubert and Carpenter, 1999). The sample selection was thought to be a clear strength of the paper.

2. **Data**: In addition to the strength of the selection of the sample, the use of interviews to obtain data is highly congruent with the study design and is another strength of the paper.

3. **Participants**: As stated above, the selection of the participants is a clear strength of the paper.

4. **Credibility**: The researchers did try to establish the credibility or authenticity of their findings and this is to the betterment of the paper. However, the use of so-called independent co-examiners to confer credibility on the interpretations of the researchers is problematic.[4]

Ethical dimensions

The section of the paper dealing with ethics was thought by the reviewers to be very strong and a clear strength of the paper. There was no evidence of breach of ethical issues (Burnard and Chapman, 2003; McHale and Gallagher, 2003). Furthermore, the reviewers felt that one of the key contributions that this paper made was to demonstrate that, if adequate and thorough safeguards are put in place, and if the research is conducted with the necessary levels of sensitivity, then research with vulnerable groups focusing on previous traumatic experiences is clearly possible without causing harm to the research participants. It is again worthy of note that none of the participants who volunteered subsequently withdrew because of being 'harmed' as a result of talking about their experiences of sexual abuse during childhood. Rather, the opposite effect was reported, namely that (Rahm *et al.*, 2006, p. 108):

> it had been of therapeutic value for them to participate in the study, and they felt it important to tell about their experiences in order to increase knowledge about sexual abuse.

---

4 We have already covered this debate in the reviews numbered 4, 6 and 17.

Interpretive dimensions

1. The discussion section focuses on providing references from the extant literature to support the findings of the current study. The findings were indeed supported by this literature, which again was not surprising, given that for the reviewers this paper was perhaps confirming what we already knew.

2. The interpretations are the results. The reviewers felt that the interpretations could have withstood additional further analysis as the findings might not be parsimonious. For example, some of the themes appeared to have conceptual overlap with one another, the themes 'feeling different' and 'feeling like an outsider' being a good illustration of this. The limitations of the study were mentioned but these were restricted to the often cited limitation regarding the non-generalisability of qualitative findings. While it appeared that the authors were referring to nomothetic generalisability here, this was not made clear.

3. As stated above, the authors draw upon existing empirical and theoretical literature to support their findings, and each of their findings finds support in the extant literature. The use of the 1971 Lewis text to support the assertion that shame is seldom dealt with in therapy appears to be a strange choice. A more contemporary reference was needed here, particularly as more recent literature indicates that attention to shame and its clinical implications has increased over recent years (see for example, Gilbert, 1998; Tangney, 2001; Tangney and Dearing, 2002).

4. No alternative explanations for the findings are mentioned.

5. As the study claims to be using a 'mainly qualitative' design (and there is clear evidence of quantitative methods in the design), it might be regarded as something of an insight that the authors do not appear to distinguish between practical and statistical significance. Indeed, even though the study in part uses quantitative methods, there is no evidence of quantitative attempts to determine the validity or reliability of the findings (Polit *et al.*, 2001).

6. There does not appear to be any evidence of generalisations made that are not warranted on the basis of the sample used.

7. The researchers offer subtle implications for P/MH nursing practice. They argue that it is a challenge for health professionals to talk about sexual abuse and the hidden aspects of shame and continue to suggest that the study may provide a way to understand some of the reactions that follow sexual abuse. However, the reviewers felt that the practice implications arising could have been much stronger. For example, the reviewers hoped that given the extent of the problem and the powerful nature of the data, it would have been very useful to consider how these dynamics 'play out' in P/MH nurse/client encounters. Similarly, it would have had utility to consider how P/MH nurses might work with these experiences and better understand the specific nature of help/support that such clients need. Only one implication for further research was identified (p. 108) and this was also regarded as a limitation. Additional research questions could

have included: what attitudes/qualities within the P/MH nurse (or mental health practitioner) appear to be useful (or harmful) in helping the client deal with the sense of shame? How/why do these qualities/attitudes work? What interventions appear to be most useful in helping the client deal with the sense of shame? Does it make a difference to the outcomes *vis à vis* shame if the self-help groups invite male victims of sexual abuse in childhood?

Presentational and stylistic dimensions

1. Given the word limit of the journal, the article contains enough information to enable a thorough critique, notwithstanding the lack of a conceptual framework.
2. The paper is reasonably well written, especially when one considers that it is written by someone who does not have English as a first language. There is no evidence of pretentious or tautological wording.
3. The report follows a logical sequence.
4. There is no evidence of unnecessary, irrelevant details.
5. Given that the report claims to be 'mainly qualitative' it is right and proper that biases are evident. A qualitative research study has to have bias; bias that is both necessary and purposeful (Morse, 1998).[5]
6. The report is written using tentative language.
7. No evidence of sexist language.
8. The reviewers felt that the title was powerful and captured something of the *essence* of the experiences being studied; this was felt to be a strength of the paper. The abstract provided an adequate summary.

The meaning of qualitative results

The reviewers felt that there were some strengths and some limitations evident in the process of analysis used in the paper. The authors stated that they used a 'mainly qualitative' method, which in and of itself, is somewhat unclear. What gave the reviewers most concern, however. was the limited depth of the analysis and the lack of evidence of the four stages of qualitative data analysis (Morse, 1994). In keeping with Morse's four stages of qualitative data analysis, high-quality qualitative research goes beyond the words, sees past the obvious, accesses the underlying and the hidden, and enlanguages the often present yet invisible process/culture/experiences (Cutcliffe and McKenna, 2004). The authors' attempts to establish the credibility of their findings have already been covered above. One further issue that gave concern to the reviewers was that the authors did not ask a question about shame and/or experiences of shame.

---

5 We have already covered this methodological issue in critique Example 4.

The importance of qualitative results

As stated previously, the reviewers feel that this area is certainly one that should be studied and better understood. What was a concern for the reviewers, however, was the issue of whether or not a qualitative method was indicated given what we already know about this phenomenon. As a result, the reviewers were left wondering whether, if a study simply reproduces that what we already know and understand reasonably well, does this mean that the results are trivial? In response to this question, the reviewers accept the axiom that there is always something of value, something to be learned from each study. Nevertheless, the reviewers felt that more illuminating questions could have been asked which would have further added to the extant knowledge base more than this study.

The transferability of qualitative results

This aspect of the findings was thought to be a strength of the paper. The details provided about the sample and the setting was thorough, as a result the context of the study was easy to understand. Accordingly, the findings appear to have idiographic generalisability to any 'case' involving sexual abuse during childhood and shame, irrespective of the particular culture, country or mental health setting.

The implications of qualitative results

As stated above, the reviewers felt that the authors of this paper had possibly missed something of an opportunity to explore the implications of this study. While Polit *et al*. (2001) advocate that the researchers can consider a range of future research, practice and/or theory development implications, these appeared to be lacking in the paper. The findings in this study are potentially powerful and illuminating and will clearly impact upon practice, yet an exploration of these practice-level implications was not evident. The reviewers wanted to know how these experiences and the resultant behaviours may be manifest in P/MH nurse/client encounters. They wanted to see evidence of the authors examining how P/MH nurses might work with these client experiences and better understand the specific nature of help/support that such clients need. The reviewers also wanted to see a range of future possible research questions, such as what attitudes/qualities within the P/MH nurse (or mental health practitioner) appear to be useful (or harmful) in helping the client deal with the sense of shame. How/why do these qualities/attitudes work? What interventions appear to be most useful in helping the client deal with the sense of shame? Does it make a difference to the outcomes *vis à vis* shame if the self-help groups invite male victims of sexual abuse in childhood? Finally, the reviewers wanted to see evidence that the authors had thought about the theoretical implications; most especially, how these new findings added to, confirmed/refuted and/or built upon our existing understanding of shame.

References

Burnard, P. and Chapman, C. (2003) *Professional and Ethical Issues in Nursing*. Baillière Tindall, Edinburgh.

Cutcliffe, J. R. and McKenna, H. P. (2004) Expert qualitative researchers and the use of audit trails. *Journal of Advanced Nursing*, **45**(2), 126–33.

Gilbert, P. (1998) What is shame? Some core issues and controversies. In: *Shame: Interpersonal Behaviour, Psychopathology and Culture* (eds. P. Gilbert and B. Andrews). Oxford University Press, Oxford.

Hasse, M. and Magnusson, L. (2005) A concept analysis of shame. In: *The Essential Concepts of Nursing* (eds. J. R. Cutcliffe and H. P. McKenna), pp. 243–56. Elsevier, London.

Kvale, S. (1996) *Interviews: An Introduction to Qualitative Research Interviewing*. Sage, Thousand Oaks.

McHale, J. and Gallagher, A. (2003) *Nursing and Human Rights*. Butterworth-Heinemann, Edinburgh.

Morse, J. M. (1994) Qualitative research: fact or fantasy? In: *Critical issues in Qualitative Health Research* (ed. J. M. Morse), pp. 1–7. Sage, London.

Morse, J. M. (1998) What's wrong with random selection? *Qualitative Health Research*, **8**(7), 733–5.

Polit, D. F., Beck, C. T. and Hungler, B. P. (2001) *Essentials of Nursing Research: Methods, Appraisal and Utilization*, 5th edn. Lippincott, Philadelphia.

Rahm, G. B., Renck, B. and Ringsberg, K. C. (2006) 'Disgust, disgust beyond description' – shame cues to detect shame in disguise, in interviews with women who were sexually abused during childhood. *Journal of Psychiatric and Mental Health Nursing*, **13**(1), 100–9.

Streubert, H. J. and Carpenter, D. R. (1999) *Qualitative Research in Nursing: Advancing the Humanistic Perspective*. Lippincott, Philadelphia.

Tangney, J. P. (2001) Constructive and destructive aspects of shame and guilt. In: *Constructive and Destructive Behaviour: Implications for Family, School and Society* (eds. A. C. Bohart and D. J. Stipkek), pp. 127–45. American Psychological Association, Washington DC.

Tangney, J. P. and Dearing, R. L. (2002) *Shame and Guilt*. Guilford Press, New York.

Strengths and limitations of Polit, Beck and Hungler's (2001) approach

Strengths

- This is a very thorough and comprehensive approach.
- It builds upon the earlier approaches and as a result has significant advantages over some of the earlier approaches, particularly in critiquing qualitative approaches.
- It appears to give consideration to most of the fundamental components that each research report should make reference to.
- It does contain some research terminology, but this is not excessive or inappropriate. However, this does necessitate the reviewer having some understanding of basic concepts and practices within research.

- If a reviewer follows and subsequently addresses each of the questions contained within each of the five dimensions, then it is very likely that the author of the research paper reviewed may learn from a critique using Polit, Beck and Hungler's critique.

- The approach clearly encourages the reviewer(s) to think about how the findings in the reviewed paper(s) may impact on nursing practice, nursing theory and future nursing research.

- The approach includes many useful and thought-provoking questions within the headings.

- The approach allows room for the data and/or argument to be introduced to support the reviewer's criticisms/observations and suggestions for improvement.

- The addition of sections/questions that refer directly to qualitative studies are a welcome addition and go some way towards generating approaches to critiquing that are designed specifically to be used with qualitative methods.

Limitations

- The approach provide lists of questions/guidelines for the interpretive and presentational dimensions, and yet does not provide lists/guidelines for the other three dimensions. It does not explain why this is the case. This leaves reviewers wondering whether Polit, Beck and Hungler are suggesting a greater 'weighting' for these dimensions? They do not appear to make this case explicitly.

- Some of the specific guidelines might be considered to be repetitive.

- As Polit, Beck and Hungler themselves point out, a critique should highlight the positive elements of a study in addition to the limitations. However, the lists of questions in the guidelines appear to usher the reviewer into considering the limitations more than the strengths.

- The addition of the qualitative-specific sections/questions, while welcome, means that the repetitive nature of this approach is even more pronounced. Questions asked within the five dimensions are repeated in the qualitative sections.

- Clearer guidance could be added which explains how the new 'qualitative' sections fit with the existing five dimensions and thus minimize any needless repetition.

- The new 'qualitative' sections/questions, while being a welcome addition, still do not include enough reference to the underpinning philosophical stance(s) of qualitative studies, and thus the methodological questions could stand further refinement.

Reference

Polit, D. F., Beck, C. T. and Hungler, B. P. (2001) *Essentials of Nursing Research: Methods, Appraisal and Utilization*, 5th edn. Lippincott, Philadelphia.

PART 3

The development of the NPNR Journal Club approach to critiquing nursing research

The need for a new approach to critiquing nursing research? The NPNR Journal Club approach

The previous chapters have highlighted that there exist a wide range of approaches to critiquing nursing research, and we have focused on six such approaches. These represent only a sample of the different models or approaches that exist within the nursing research literature. The previous chapters have also indicated some of the strengths and limitations of these approaches.

The authors of this book would argue that there is no one, singular 'best' way to critique nursing research, and we would also argue that no one, singular model or approach will suit every nurse. Perhaps there would be merit in nurses trying out a variety of models or approaches until they find one that they feel comfortable with. Alternatively, maybe there is merit in nurses developing approaches for themselves and consequently feeling empowered by such a development. With such a possibility in mind, members of the NPNR Journal Club sampled and subsequently tried out the approaches highlighted in this book and came to the following conclusions.

1. Each of the approaches appears to have strengths and limitations. However, the following criticisms could be levelled at each of the approaches (to a greater or lesser extent). (*Note*: Especially the earlier approaches.)
2. The approaches appeared to be orientated towards (or influenced by) quantitative methods rather than qualitative methods, and appeared to be critiquing the study according to quantitative criteria rather than qualitative criteria. As indicated previously, nursing research has a history of being influenced by the medical profession (Pearson, 1992), and consequently the philosophical, epistemological and methodological beliefs of the biomedical model have been adopted by some nurse researchers. Consequently, positivistic philosophies, quantitative methods and the hegemony of the Randomised Controlled Trial (RCT) can be seen throughout many nursing research reports. Given such an influence, it is perhaps no surprise that approaches to critiquing nursing research also reflect this 'quantitative' favouritism or leaning.
3. Nevertheless there is a growing recognition of the need to embrace qualitative research methods within nursing research (Leininger, 1992; Mueser *et*

al., 1998; Fenton, 2000; Burnard and Hannigan, 2000; Florence *et al.*, 2006; Roen *et al.*, 2006; Pluye *et al.*, 2006); hence the movement towards a more pluralistic approach, and concurrently a need for approaches to critiquing nursing research to mirror this movement towards qualitative studies. Thus approaches should be able to facilitate an adequate critique of a qualitative research study.[1]

4. The approaches appear to judge the studies according to the degree to which the results are generalisable. Whilst this may be entirely appropriate for some studies, it may not be appropriate for all of them.

5. Perhaps the approaches don't emphasise enough the need for the reviewer to consider the key practice issues that arise out of the study. That is, given that nursing is a practice-orientated discipline, ultimately the research should have some implications (or potential impact) on practice (McKenna, 2005).

The authors of this book would argue that for a model of critiquing nursing research to be comprehensive and useful, it needs to consider the theoretical, methodological, ethical substantive and presentational issues. Additionally, we would wholeheartedly agree with the view that critiques must emphasise *both* the strengths and limitations of the research. However, because nursing is a 'practice led' discipline, we would argue that additional criteria for judging models or approaches for critiquing nursing research might include the following questions:

1. Is it easily understandable by and accessible to nurses? Or does the extent of excessive jargon or terminology discourage the reviewer from reading the paper? (We acknowledge that there is a need for methodological clarity and precision, and accordingly the use of some terminology. Nevertheless, too much jargon/terminology within research reports is often cited as a reason for nurses not utilising the study in clinical practice.)

2. Does the model/approach to critiquing help nurses decide whether or not the research makes a difference to their practice?

3. Does the model/approach to critiquing help nurses decide whether or not the research has *potential* to make a difference to practice?

4. What are the key points that arise from the study; in particular, the key points for practice?

5. Does the model/approach to critiquing necessitate the need for a PhD, MSc or a BSc degree in order to be able to make sense of the critique and subsequently the research?

---

1 *Footnote to the 2nd edn*: While there is evidence of some progression towards this position, an examination of the relevant extant literature suggests that there is certainly room for additional work. Along with developing methods to combine qualitative studies into some meta-syntheses, this remains one of the most pressing issues facing nursing epistemologists and theorists.

We would argue that the approach developed by the NPNR Journal Club perhaps addresses some of these issues, and furthermore, *is an approach developed by nurses, for nurses, out of a need to do so*. The approach attempts not only to comment on the reviewed paper, but also to locate arguments, issues and questions within broader contexts, be they larger 'policy' contexts (see increased use of evidence-based practice, Chapter 6), or practice context (see experiences of violence, Chapter 10), or methodological contexts (see methodological issues in measuring attitudes, Chapter 9). Consequently, an individual reading one of the NPNR Journal Club-style critiques not only hopefully gains a sense of the paper's strengths and limitations, but additionally is directed to relevant, linked material that supports the critique and leads the reviewer in the direction of some of the associated literature. This enables the reviewer (and the author of the paper reviewed) to become better informed on the matters raised.

We suggest therefore, that some of the emerging strengths/features of the NPNR Journal Club approach to critiquing might include the following:

- It asks: how does the reviewed piece of work effect/help/benefit you as a clinician, educationalist, researcher or manager?
- The inclusion of three key points for each reviewed paper.
- The approach can be used for both qualitative and quantitative research.
- It urges the reviewer to consider: what meaning or worth does the study have for the practice and knowledge base of P/MH nursing?
- It urges the reviewers to reference their criticisms/points raised, and this hopefully raises the level of academic debate.
- It urges the reviewers to consider the paper in a 'holistic' rather than 'reductionist' manner. It urges reviewers to consider each of these identified sections separately and as part of the 'whole'.
- It embraces the notion of evolutionary/developmental approaches to critiquing research. Thus the approach is not static and can evolve over time, aggregating reviewers' confidence in the approach as it is used.

As with the introduction of any new practice (Ward *et al.*, 1998), the introduction of a new approach to critiquing research takes time for the practitioners to feel 'at ease' and familiar with. In the early stages of such an introduction, practitioners perhaps lack confidence in the new approach/new practice, until they can experience the benefits for themselves. Importantly, in the early days of the Journal Club, we adopted the empowering philosophy of practice development described by Ward *et al.* (1998) to facilitate the uptake of the Journal Club's approach to critiquing research. Consequently, it was emphasised to each Journal Club, that the approach was developmental. It could and indeed, should, evolve over time, in direct response to the members' feedback, derived from their experience of using the approach. Thus, reviews produced during the 'early days' of the Journal Club perhaps are less comprehensive, less extensive

---

Box 9.1 Guidelines of the NPNR Journal Club approach to critiquing nursing research

1. Follow the sequence of the paper as laid out by the author(s).
2. Consider each of the theoretical, substantive, methodological, ethical and presentational dimensions for each of the sections (headings) identified by the paper's author.
3. Consider each of these identified sections separately and as part of the 'whole', since individually well-written sections may not necessarily add up to become a cumulative whole. This minimises the sense of reductionism present in most critiquing approaches.
4. Ask methodological questions in keeping with the design/paradigm identified by the author.
5. Draw upon any existing approach to critiquing for specific questions if you feel these add to your critique.
6. Locate the questions/issues you raise in your critique within the broader practice, education, research and policy literature.
7. Reflect on and identify how the reviewed piece of work affects/helps/ benefits you as a clinician, educationalist, researcher or manager.
8. Reflect on and identify the meaning or worth that the study has for the practice and knowledge base of P/MH nursing.
9. Identify three key points, of which at least one is positive and one negative.
10. Do ensure that you look for, and highlight, at least one strength of the paper. It is all too easy to overemphasise the negative.
11. Provide references to substantiate your critique.

---

and less expansive than later reviews. Concomitantly, the members' confidence in the critiques they produced, also increased over time, as they became more familiar with the approach, felt more involved with its development, and saw their reviews published.

References

Burnard, P. and Hannigan, B. (2000) Qualitative and quantitative approaches in nursing: moving the debate forward. *Journal of Psychiatric and Mental Health Nursing*, **7**(4), 363–70.

Florence, Z., Schulz, T. and Pearson, A. (recovered 2006) Inter-reviewer agreement: an analysis of the degree to which agreement occurs when using tools for the appraisal, extraction and meta-synthesis of qualitative research findings. *The Cochrane Collaboration.* http://www.cochrane.org/colloquia/abstracts/melbourne/O-69.htm.

Leininger, M. (1992) Current issues, problems and trends to advance qualitative paradigmatic research methods for the future. *Qualitative Health Research*, **2**(4), 392–415.

McKenna, H. P. (2005) Research outputs, environment and esteem. *Journal of Research in Nursing*, **10**, 597–600.

Pearson, A. (1992) Knowing nursing: emerging paradigms in nursing. *Knowledge for Nursing Practice* (eds. K. Robinson and B. Vaughan), pp. 213–26. Butterworth-Heinemann, Oxford.

Pluye, P., Grad, R., Dunikowski, L. and Stephenson, R. (recovered 2006) A challenging mixed literature review experience web site address

Roen, K., Rodgers, R., Arai, L., Petticrew, M., Popay, J., Roberts, H. and Sowden, H. (recovered 2006) Narrative synthesis of qualitative and quantitative evidence: an analysis of tools and techniques web reference. http://www.cochrane.org/colloquia/abstracts/ottawa/O-058.htm

Ward, M., Titchen, A., Morell, C., McCormack, B. and Kitson, A. (1998) Using a supervisory framework to support and evaluate a multiproject practice development programme. *Journal of Clinical Nursing*, **7**, 29–36.

The first phase of Journal Club development: early attempts

Example 11: The NPNR National Journal Club: review from the 2nd meeting

The paper reviewed was Scanlon, C. and Wier, W. S. (1997) Learning from practice: mental health nurses' perceptions and experiences of clinical supervision. *Journal of Advanced Nursing*, **26**, 295–303.

Abstract/overview

This paper reports on a small-scale qualitative study which attempted to explore P/MH nurses' perceptions and experiences of clinical supervision. The authors conducted a series of semi-structured interviews, analysed the data, and found encouraging early indicators that P/MH nurses are becoming better able to reflect upon their formative learning needs, and so take seriously their need for professional support, as they strive towards therapeutic relationships with clients. The authors discovered evidence that suggests 'good enough supervision' was the exception rather than the rule.

Introduction

Feedback comments indicated that members felt that each of the three questions identified within the introduction were worthy of investigation in their own right. Furthermore, comments indicated that members felt that the purposes of the study were indicated in the research questions. However, it was not clear whether the study was intended to induce a theory where no current theory existed or to add to knowledge and understanding that already exists.

Literature review

Feedback comments indicated that members felt that this paper, like many papers on clinical supervision, lacked a complete representation of all that supervision can be. Additionally, while it is appropriate to discuss parallel processes within supervision, certainly if one uses a psychodynamic model (Hawkins and Shohet, 1996), members felt that it was not appropriate to describe all clinical supervisor/supervisee relationships in terms of parallel processes.

Research design: sample

While some reservations were raised concerning the size of the sample, it was acknowledged that relatively small samples can still provide rich data for qualitative studies (Streubert and Carpenter, 1999). However, concerns were raised concerning the composition of the sample. Whilst purposeful sampling is entirely appropriate with the qualitative method advocated (Morse, 1991; Cassell, 2004), it was felt that a little more effort could have gone into obtaining the sample rather than the convenience sample used. Reed et al. (1996), for example, argue that the research question and methods used dictate the need for a sample that is relevant to the theoretical development within the study. To limit this sample to nurses who were known to the researchers perhaps imposes unnecessary limitations and may well have had an impact on the richness of the data gathered.

Research design: data collection

Comments indicated that members felt that the method of data collection was appropriate. Another point of view argued that since the researchers were concerned with obtaining the 'lived experiences' of P/MH nurses who receive clinical supervision, it might have been more appropriate to have used a phenomenological approach (Heidegger, 1962; Walters, 1995; Van Manen, 1997). More detail was necessary, for example, about what type of qualitative approach was used and why? Were other approaches considered? Therefore the paper might have been better for having more detail in some areas.

Ethical considerations

The paper appeared to lack information on ethical issues, e.g. did anyone *not* consent to take part?

Data analysis

Feedback comments indicated that members felt that while the methods appeared to be appropriate, it was not clear how the development of the emergent themes was achieved. Consequently, members were left wondering if there had been some slurring of the methodology (Baker *et al.*, 1992) and what influence this might have had on the results. The use of interviewee statements was felt to be particularly useful not only in terms of establishing the credibility of the findings but also adding to the understanding of the emerging theory. Efforts appear to have been made to ensure the rigour of the data analysis. However, importing such terms and methods that were developed for quantitative methods, such as 'inter-rater reliability', was felt to be inappropriate for this study (Cutcliffe and McKenna, 1999).

Results, discussion and conclusions

The results section contained some valuable themes, and these themes are supported by previous studies (Bishop, 1994; Fowler, 1995; Severinsson, 1995; Butterworth *et al.*, 1997). While in response to the results the authors make some useful comments in the discussion section, it might have been worthwhile to expand the implications for their findings to include issues such as training/education in clinical supervision.

Final comments: what meaning does this have for psychiatric and mental health nurses?

The key points raised from the review of this paper are listed in Table 9.1. Few would dispute that the practice and evaluation of clinical supervision continue to be important issues for nurses, and the continued interest in the subject is reflected in the number of articles in the nursing literature that feature supervision. It is also reasonable to suggest that there remain many unanswered questions. Therefore any attempt to examine these issues and address these questions appears to have merit. Since, within the substantive area, there remain epistemological questions – questions concerning the process and questions concerning the outcomes and efficacy – there is a clear need to conduct both qualitative and quantitative enquiries. The contribution of qualitative studies should not be ignored, even though there is growing pressure from some managers to discover a direct correlation between receiving clinical supervision and improved client care.

However, while this paper does add evidence to certain current arguments, e.g. the problems and difficulties of having a direct line manager as your supervisor, and the distinct lack of specific supervision training that individuals have had, it does not appear to be saying a great deal that is new. Perhaps it would have been more worthwhile to focus on these identified problems and either investigate them more fully qualitatively (e.g. how do the problems of having a direct line manager as a supervisor affect the process of supervision?). Or perhaps they should have been investigated quantitatively to find out how many individuals have encountered the problems (e.g. how many of the nurses receive supervision from their direct line manager?). Such studies might then provide a deeper, more complete understanding of the extent of the problem.

Table 9.1 Key points arising from review No. 2.

1. The article reflected a current and important theme within P/MH nursing – clinical supervision as a vehicle for improving practice – and attempts to explore and evaluate clinical supervision should be supported.

2. Members were not convinced that the paper was saying anything new, while it did add weight to certain arguments (e.g. not having a manager as your supervisor).

3. The limitations of the sampling strategy may have had an impact on the results.

The last issue, that of sampling strategies, is relevant to all nursing research studies. The results presented in this study, as with any research study, are only as credible as the methodology allows (Polit and Hungler, 1997; Polit *et al.*, 2001). Practitioners concerned with conducting studies that would either support or refute the practice of clinical supervision need to consider methodological and sampling issues. In this instance there may have been merit in sampling all P/MH nurses from one clinical area, or one particular grade. While any theory induced would only be pertinent to that clinical area studied or group of individuals, each microcosm of nursing bears a resemblance to nursing as a whole. As Denzin and Lincoln (1994, p. 201) state:

> Every instance of a case or process bears the general class of phenomena it belongs to. However, any given instance is likely to be particular and unique.

Therefore, while the authors would not be able to generalise the experiences of clinical supervision described, there might well be elements of the theory that all nurses recognise as having meaning for themselves and can relate to their own practice and experience of clinical supervision.

References

Baker, C., Weust, J. and Stern, P. N. (1992) Method slurring: the grounded theory/phenomenology example. *Journal of Advanced Nursing*, **17**, 1355–60.

Bishop, V. (1994) Clinical supervision questionnaire. *Nursing Times*, **90**(48), 40–2.

Butterworth, T., Carson, J., White, E., Jeacock, J., Clements, A. and Bishop, V. (1997) *It Is Good to Talk. Clinical Supervision and Mentorship. An Evaluation Study in England and Scotland*. The School of Nursing, Midwifery and Health Visiting, The University of Manchester.

Cassell, C. (2004) *Essential Guide to Qualitative Methods in Organizational Research*. Sage, London.

Cutcliffe, J. R. and McKenna, H. P. (1999) Establishing the credibility of qualitative research findings: the plot thickens. *Journal of Advanced Nursing*, **30**(2), 374–80.

Denzin, N. K. and Lincoln, Y. S. (1994) Entering the field of qualitative research In: *Handbook of Qualitative Research* (eds. N. K. Denzin and Y. S. Lincoln), pp. 1–17. Sage, London.

Fowler, J. (1995) Nurses' perceptions of the elements of good supervision. *Nursing Times*, **91**(22), 33–7.

Hawkins, P. and Shohet, R. (1996) *Supervision in the Helping Professions*. Open University Press, Milton Keynes.

Heidegger, M. (1962) *Being and Time*. Harper & Row, New York.

Morse, J. M. (1991) Strategies for sampling. In: *Qualitative Nursing Research: A Contemporary Dialogue* (ed. J. M. Morse), pp. 127–45. Sage, London.

Polit, D. F. and Hungler, B. P. (1997) *Essentials of Nursing Research: Methods, Appraisal and Utilization*, 4th edn. Lippincott, Philadelphia.

Polit, D. F., Beck, C. T. and Hungler, B. P. (2001) *Essentials of Nursing Research: Methods, Appraisal and Utilization*, 5th edn. Lippincott, Philadelphia.

Reed, J., Procter, S. and Murray, S. (1996) A sampling strategy for qualitative research. *Nurse Researcher*, **3**(4), 52–69.

Severinsson, E. I. (1995) The phenomenon of clinical supervision within psychiatric health care. *Journal of Psychiatric and Mental Health Nursing*, **2**, 301–9.

Streubert, H. J. and Carpenter, D. R. (1999) *Qualitative Research in Nursing: Advancing the Humanistic Perspective*. Lippincott, Philadelphia.

Van Manen, M. (1997) *Researching Lived Experience: Human Science for Action Sensitive Pedagogy*. State University of New York Press, New York.

Walters, A. J. (1995) The phenomenological movement: implications for nursing research. *Journal of Advanced Nursing*, **22**, 791–9.

Example 12: The NPNR National Journal Club: review from the 3rd meeting

The paper reviewed was Willets, L. and Leff, J. (1997) Expressed emotion and schizophrenia: the efficacy of a staff training programme. *Journal of Advanced Nursing*, **26**, 1125–33.

Abstract/overview

This paper reports on an investigation of the presence of expressed emotion (EE) in five community care facilities. The authors discovered that levels of high EE existed in some staff–client relationships. A training programme was subsequently developed to enable community mental health workers to increase their knowledge about schizophrenia and repertoire of strategies for managing a variety of difficulties. It was hoped that this training would decrease levels of EE present in their relationships with clients. The authors report a small but non-significant increase in knowledge following the training, and an increase in the use of strategies aimed at effecting change. They also report that no significant changes in EE levels were reported.

Title

Feedback comments indicated that members felt that the title could have been clearer in identifying a nursing interest. Perhaps if the title had indicated specifically which staff the training was for, it would have added to the clarity.

Abstract

Feedback comments indicated that members felt that the abstract identified the research problem, but did not specify a hypothesis or outline the methodology. Members also acknowledged that the abstract identified the major findings of the report. Concerns were also raised regarding the term 'high expressed emotion' and members felt this was a rather pejorative expression. What would it mean as a member of a family that is labelled 'high EE?'. Similarly, what affects would it have on a single (or several) member of staff to be given this label? In the same way that concerns have been raised regarding assigning labels to clients (Clunn, 1993; Thompson et al., 1988), perhaps clinicians and researchers should consider the possible deleterious effects of giving such labels to family carers or members of staff.

Introduction

Members felt that the introduction and literature review were merged, and consequently they struggled to easily identify the point the authors were trying to make. The aims of the study are clear, but it was felt that the research question could have been clearer. This was due to the terminology used. For example, the terms 'appropriate intervention strategies' and 'problematic behaviours' were thought to be somewhat ambiguous.

Literature review

The literature review included appropriate and relevant literature relating to expressed emotion; however, there appeared to be important omissions. A particular oversight was that of Brooker and Butterworth's (1991) study which described the effect on the role and function of the community psychiatric nurse (CPN) after training to deliver psychosocial intervention to families caring for a relative at home. Also not considered was Nolan et al.'s (1997) work on family care, which (amongst other issues) discusses the longitudinal nature of family care.

Members also questioned whether one could measure EE within staff in the same way as families. Although staff may be in a position so that they are part of the same community as the clients, their relationship is very different from that of the family. (For example, they leave that environment and go home to their own families.)

Method

Members stated that they felt that in places the method and introduction were merged and subsequently lacked clarity. Additionally, the strengths and weaknesses of the chosen approach were not explored. Criticisms were levelled regarding the author's reference to the limited value of naturalistic studies. Many authors, such as Lincoln and Guba (1985), Denzin and Lincoln (1994), Heidegger (1962), and Melia

(1982) would construct rigorous arguments for studying people in their natural settings. Indeed, obtaining clients' views and the lived experiences of staff caring for these people could have produced useful and valuable data, particularly as ultimately it is their care we are interested in.

Sample selection

Some reservations were raised concerning the size of the sample, although it should be noted that the authors did acknowledge this limitation. The major concern raised by members regarding the sample was what effect self-selection and the use of a convenience sample might have had on the results (Burns and Grove, 1993; Peat, 2002; Hicks, 2004). In order to enhance the validity of the findings (Polit et al., 2001; Hicks, 2004), the authors could have made some effort to include a control group, perhaps randomly selecting some of the community care staff and not providing them with the training.

Ethical considerations

There was no indication of the members of staff consenting to participate in this study. It may have been felt that staff did not need to consent, but members expressed an opinion that this was inappropriate. In terms of ethical considerations, members of staff should be treated no differently from clients (Lipson, 1994; Department of Health, 2001; McHale and Gallagher, 2003). The absence of any ethical considerations was felt to be an oversight.

Results

Members felt that the results could have been presented more clearly. For example, the tables were not properly identified in the text nor properly labelled. There was perhaps an over-zealous use of percentages for small numbers of subjects in the study.

Data analysis

On the whole the approach to data analysis appeared to be appropriate, yet some members felt that the statistical analysis was not clearly indicated. The small sample did not allow sufficient analysis (e.g. there were an insignificant number of subjects for a paired t-test; Peat (2002), Hicks (2004)) or to determine whether or not significant differences were attributable to variations in other relevant variables.

Discussion, conclusions and recommendations

Feedback comments indicated that members felt that in this section there were a number of variables which should have been clearly identified from previous studies and that had not been controlled in any way in this study. Perhaps a more useful study would have been for the authors to investigate how the course affected the practitioners' thoughts and feelings and subsequent practice of this particular client group.

Members did state that the paper highlighted some interesting lines of enquiry for possible future enquiries. One such line of enquiry would be to conduct a participation observation study of the practice of the practitioners in order to provide a further source of data. Since in this current study all the data was obtained by interviews and questionnaires and thus is provided by the practitioners, this third form of data would enable a triangulation of data and thus have the potential to add to the validity of the findings (Nolan and Behi, 1995; Begley, 1997). The conclusions might be considered to be rather assertive given the size of the sample, and members felt that the conclusions drawn did not have the evidence to support them.

Final comments: what meaning does this have for psychiatric and mental health nurses?

Some criticisms were levelled concerning how this research bridges the 'theory–practice gap' and how the results were going to aid nurses in their practice. Perhaps this reiterates the issue of the danger of research being published in journals that are read only by other researchers, and as a consequence practice remains largely unaffected by these studies – a point highlighted by Professor McKenna at the NPNR 1997 Edinburgh conference, when he stated:

> It is better that one nurse implements research findings that produce a positive effect on the quality of care, than a dozen non-cumulative research studies which end up gathering dust on a shelf.

A major issue that arose was that of researchers and practitioners having a dogmatic view of:

- (A) conditions such as schizophrenia and the care associated with people given this diagnosis, and
- (B) approaches to researching and understanding care issues for this group of people.

For example, Gournay (1996) advocates adopting a more biologically oriented approach to caring for individuals termed to be 'schizophrenic' and that disorders, such as schizophrenia, will become clear beyond ambiguity in our lifetime. Other authors highlight that psychosocial intervention for these clients and their families is the way forward (Gamble *et al.*, 1994). Whereas other authors have suggested that case management provides answers to some of the problems of providing care for these clients and their families (Ford *et al.*, 1995). However Moorey (1998) draws attention to the number of recent reviews of a large body of evidence which cast considerable doubt on the reliability, construct validity, predictive validity and aetiological specificity of the diagnosis of schizophrenia. Questions concerned with the cause and treatment of schizophrenia, and the value of interventions for people with this label then become incoherent if the notion of schizophrenia is rejected as a meaningful scientific construct (Moorey, 1998).

Strict adherence to one particular approach to providing care at the expense of all other approaches appears to drastically limit the care options available to client and practitioner. Similarly, to restrict the focus of research to such a narrow subject area when understanding is far from complete appears somewhat premature. This narrow-mindedness appears all the more inappropriate given other author's statements regarding the continued uncertainty surrounding care of such people. Dawson (1997, p. 1) makes this point most clearly when he states

> The truth of the matter is that we are now as far removed from such a theory as we were 20 or 30 years ago. We have not the faintest notion of what might be occurring in the brain... that is we do not yet have a model of normal thought processes, let alone 'abnormal' thought processes.

Opinion was divided regarding the readability of the paper, with some members reporting that they found this to be an interesting and thought-provoking paper. Members also stated that they wondered if the authors had tried to accomplish too much with one study, in that it appeared that the authors were concerned with both evaluating the training course they provided and simultaneously examining change in EE and the change in interaction that this may produce.

Table 9.2 Key points arising from review No. 3.

1. As laudable as any nursing related research study may be, if it ultimately makes no difference to the care of clients, then how valuable and useful is it?

2. Wholesale adoption of one particular approach to providing care at the expense of all other approaches is at best restrictive and limiting and at worst damaging and deleterious.

3. Similarly, wholesale adoption of one particular research paradigm to the exclusion of others can only limit the depth of understanding available to the researcher and force him/her to view the world through a particular lens.

References

Begley, C. M. (1996) Using triangulation in nursing research. *Journal of Advanced Nursing*, **24**, 122–8.

Brooker, C. and Butterworth, T. (1991) Working with families caring for a relative with schizophrenia: the evolving role of the community psychiatric nurse. *International Journal of Nursing Studies*, **28**(2), 189–200.

Burns, N. and Grove, S. K. (1993) *The Practice of Nursing Research: Conduct, Critique and Utilisation*, 2nd edn. W. B. Saunders, Philadelphia.

Clunn, P. A. (1993) The child. In: *Mental Health – Psychiatric Nursing* (eds. R. P. Rawlings, F. R. Williams and C. K. Beck), pp. 715–48. C. V. Mosby, St Louis.

Dawson, P. J. (1997) A reply to Kevin Gournay's 'Schizophrenia: a review of the contemporary literature and implications for mental health nursing theory, practice and education'. *Journal of Psychiatric and Mental Health Nursing*, **4**, 1–7.

Denzin, N. K. and Lincoln, Y. S. (1994) Entering the field of qualitative research. In: *A Handbook of Qualitative Research* (eds. N. K. Denzin and Y. S. Lincoln), pp. 1–17. Sage, California.

Department of Health (2001) *Research Governance Framework for Health and Social Care*. HMSO, London.

Fenton, W. S. (2000) Evolving perspectives on individual psychotherapy for schizophrenia. *Schizophrenia Bulletin*, **26**, 47–72.

Ford, R., Beadsmore, A., Ryan, P., Repper, J., Craig, J. and Muijen, M. (1995) Providing a safety net: case mangement for people with a serious mental illness. *Journal of Mental Health*, **1**, 91–7.

Gamble, C., Midence, K. and Leff, J. (1994) The effects of family work training on mental health nurses' attitude to and knowledge of schizophrenia: a replication. *Journal of Advanced Nursing*, **19**, 1169–77.

Gournay, K. (1996) Schizophrenia: a review of the contemporary literature and implications for mental health nursing theory, practice and education. *Journal of Psychiatric and Mental Health Nursing*, **3**, 7–12.

Heidegger, M. (1962) *Being and Time*. Harper & Row, New York.

Hicks, C. (2004) *Research Methods for Clinical Therapists: Applied Project Design and Analysis*. Churchill Livingstone, Edinburgh.

Lincoln, Y. S. and Guba, E. G. (1985) *Naturalistic Enquiry*. Sage, Newbury Park, CA.

Lipson, J. G. (1994) Ethical issues in ethnography. In: *Critical Issues in Qualitative Research Methods* (eds. J. M. Morse), pp. 333–55. Sage, London.

McHale, J. and Gallagher, A. (2003) *Nursing and Human Rights*. Butterworth-Heinemann, Edinburgh.

Melia, K. M. (1982) 'Tell it as it is' – qualitative methodology and nursing research: understanding the student nurse's world. *Journal of Advanced Nursing*, **7**, 327–35.

Moorey, J. (1998) The ethics of professionalised care. In: *Psychiatric Nursing: Ethical Strife* (eds. P. Barker and B. Davidson). Arnold, London.

Mueser, K., Bond, G., Drake, R. *et al.* (1998) Models of community care for severe mental illness: a review of research on case management. *Schizophrenia Bulletin*, **24**, 37–74.

Nolan, M. and Behi, R. (1995) Triangulation: the best of all worlds? *British Journal of Nursing*, **4**(14), 829–32.

Nolan, M., Grant, G. and Keady, J. (1997) *Understanding Family Care: the Multi-dimensional Nature of Caring and Coping*. Open University Press, Oxford.

Peat, J. (2002) *Health Science Research: a Handbook of Quantitative Methods*. Sage, London.

Pluye, P., Grad, R., Dunikowski, L. and Stephenson, R. (recovered 2006) A challenging mixed literature review experience. *12th Cochrane Colloquium*, The International Cochrane Collaboration, Ottawa. http://cochrane.mcmaster.ca/ottcolloquium.asp.

Polit, D. F., Beck, C. T. and Hungler, B. P. (2001) *Essentials of Nursing Research: Methods, Appraisal and Utilization*, 5th edn. Lippincott, Philadelphia.

Thompson, I. E., Melia, K. M. and Boyd, K. (1988) *Nursing Ethics*. Churchill Livingstone, Edinburgh.

CHAPTER 10

The second stage of the NPNR Journal Club development: taking shape

Example 13: The NPNR National Journal Club: review from the 4th meeting

The paper reviewed was Repper, J., Ford, R. and Cooke, A. (1994) How can nurses build trusting relationships with people who have severe and long-term mental health problems? Experiences of case managers and their clients. *Journal of Advanced Nursing*, **19**, 1096–104.

Abstract/overview

This paper reports on a study that investigated how case managers who worked specifically with people with long-term mental health problems formed and maintained relationships with their clients. The authors conducted 46 in-depth interviews with these case managers and their clients, and using a qualitative method, analysed the interview data and produced a framework of themes. They argued that these themes revealed how both clients and case managers focused on the problems and strategies of forming and maintaining relationships. Furthermore, they suggested that case managers adopted a philosophy that enabled both parties to feel positive about the work.

Title

Feedback comments indicated that members felt that even though the paper is five years old, the paper remains topical and has an appropriate focus and that that this was reflected in the title.

Abstract

Members felt that the abstract introduced the focus of the study, gave a very brief outline of the method and identified the major findings of the report. Concerns were raised regarding the imprecision of the description of the qualitative methodology. Perhaps a summary of the central themes would have enhanced the abstract.

Introduction

The introduction was felt to include the appropriate background to the study, and a rationale for undertaking the study. Perhaps this section could have been enhanced by including operational definitions of terms such as 'trusting relationship'. Also, it was unclear whether the American definition of 'case management' was adopted as the operational definition for this study. Another argument stated that with this paper being published in an international journal, the authors might have benefited from setting the context of the history of case management in the UK.

The method

Members stated that they felt that the method had several weaknesses. While alternative data collection methods were considered, members argued that the strengths and weaknesses of the chosen approach were not explored in enough detail. A stronger argument could have been constructed drawing on the extensive literature that refers to the value of naturalistic studies (Heidegger, 1962; Melia, 1982; Lincoln and Guba, 1985; Benner and Wrubel, 1989; Denzin and Lincoln, 1994), particularly given the need to uncover the knowledge embedded in the clinical experience of the case managers and the 'lived experiences' of the clients themselves (Benner, 1984; Benner and Wrubel, 1989; Walters, 1995; Van Manen, 1997). Criticisms were also levelled regarding the incomplete review of the literature. The authors made reference to 'previous studies' without citing these specifically, nor did they include any critique of these studies.

Sample selection

Members raised concerns regarding the nature of the sampling strategy. The case managers' influence on sample selection is likely to have affected the results, and members wondered if this amounted to a form of internal censorship. While the authors acknowledge this limitation and state they will account for the bias by marking quotations from this group with an asterisk, no asterisk is to be found on any of the quotations. It appears that the authors used purposeful sampling (Patton, 1990; Morse, 1991; Streubert and Carpenter, 1999) yet they do not make this specific, nor do they identify the minimum criteria for inclusion in this sample.

Members' feedback indicated that they would have liked to have heard more from the clients. Certain clients were excluded from providing any data at the behest of some case managers and the reasons for this exclusion were highlighted. This desire to see more data from the clients warrants further consideration. Until 1985 relatively little research had been conducted to elicit the views of users of mental health services (McIver, 1991a,b). Researchers appeared to have a concern that the nature of mental illness precluded users of the services from having the ability to express valid and reliable opinions. Arguments suggested that if the user has a distorted state of mind, how can they offer reliable opinions of their service? The case managers may have had similar concerns. However, more recently attempts have been made to obtain the views of mental health service users (MIND, 1986; Elbeck and Fecteau, 1990; Elzinga and Barlow, 1991; Sheppard, 1993; Pickett et al., 1993; Babiker and Thorne, 1993; Lovell, 1995; Stephenson et al., 1995; Beech and Norman, 1995; Mental Health Foundation, 2000). Therefore the members' argument in favour of wishing to see more data from the clients appears to be well founded.

Ethical considerations

The absence of any ethical considerations or details regarding ethical approval was felt to be an oversight (Lipson, 1994; McHale and Gallagher, 2003; Burnard and Chapman, 2003). The paper contained no mention of ethical considerations, neither those pertaining to the staff nor those to the clients. Members were left wondering whether any clients refused to be interviewed, and if so, why?

Data analysis

Members' feedback indicated that they felt the data analysis section lacked detail. The paper is somewhat imprecise with regard to the research design, in that it appears to be using a phenomenological method yet does not make this clear. However, the major criticism of this section was the lack of a comprehensive explanation of how the themes were induced. Members wanted to see how the researchers had moved from labels (initial categorisation) to condensing these into 'main problem areas' to the central themes. Additionally, it would have been useful to see how the themes/ categorisations interrelated with one another.

Findings

Members wondered if the findings and the discussion of the findings had been amalgamated into one section. However, points of view were raised that argued in favour of a more in-depth discussion of the findings. For example, when the authors highlighted the practice of adopting certain perspectives and having understanding and empathy, members wanted to know how the case managers adopted these perspectives? How did they convey this empathy? How did the clients experience it? It should be noted that on the whole the members felt that the findings reflected their understanding of the practice and sentiments of case management. Members also stated that the findings were somewhat obvious, but this does not mean they were not valuable.

Discussion, conclusions and recommendations

Members did state that while the conclusions were somewhat generalised, the paper highlighted some interesting lines of enquiry for possible future studies. The addition of some recommendations arising from the findings might have been useful.

Final comments: what meaning does this have for psychiatric and mental health nurses?

Few P/MH nurses would argue with the findings of this study regarding the formation of relationships. Establishing a trusting relationship, engaging clients and communicating with clients have been identified as integral aspects of psychiatric nursing in many studies. For example, the review of psychiatric nursing in 1994 (Department of Health, 1994), reaffirmed the idea of what P/MH nurses should be doing and summarised these activities under the following headings:

- establishing therapeutic relationships resting in a respect for others
- responding flexibly to changing patient needs
- making risk assessments and judgements

As long ago as the 1970s Towell's (1975) study identified several roles for P/MH nurses in different clinical settings, including having a significant role in treatment within therapeutic communities. Cormack (1983) found that psychiatric staff were effective at, amongst other activities, staff-initiated interactions. More recently, Duffy and Lee (1998) found that the core activities of P/MH nurses within contemporary trusts included psychosocial interventions and therapies.

Hill and Michael (1996) used a phenomenological approach and found that a core activity of psychiatric nurses is their ordinary contact which is respectful and empathic. Similarly, Gallop (1997) has suggested

> the potential power of psychiatric nursing comes from the unique nature of the caring relationship

and the uniqueness is centred on the use of empathy, whereby the nurse comes to know and understand the world of the other and to use that understanding constructively. Consequently, while few P/MH nurses would disagree with the findings, is the paper under review saying anything new? Is it adding to the understanding or is it simply confirming current understanding? The paper appeared to have the potential to explore these activities and processes in more detail, and this would have added to the extent of the knowledge.

The paper also appears to be saying that it is easy to work with clients with severe and long-term mental health problems, and this may not always be the case. The sometimes complex process of forming ordinary relationships with extra-ordinary people is not always a simple matter (Hill and Michael, 1996). Again, perhaps this complexity could have been explored more fully if the researchers had included more detail. For example, a dynamic of any P/MH nurse (including case managers)/client relationship is the extent to which the nurses are prepared to exercise power over clients or to share power with clients (Campbell, 1998). Therefore crucial questions should be asked regarding issues such as how does the case manager abdicate this potential power to the client and yet at the same time reconcile this practice with the possibility of having to force hospital admission and/or treatment on the client? Such endeavours to maintain the equilibrium and symmetry of power dynamics cannot be easy, particularly when both parties are aware of the potential for the use of power by the case manager as a form of intervention. It is conceivably the situations where major problems occur in forming relationships that reveal most about the complexity of this process. However, there was an absence of such situations within the paper.

It is reasonable to suggest that problems can exist regarding engagement for all clients, not just for the client group featured in this study. Given the qualitative nature of the study, the authors are not attempting to generalise their findings to a wider population, but they do state (p. 1104):

> there are others for whom the approach and strategies identified in this study offer useful guidelines for their work

Consequently, the paper can be considered to be brave as it invites others to come on board and debate and discuss. Therefore it can be considered to be valuable and relevant to all.

Table 10.1 Key points arising from review No. 4.

1. It is a motivational paper and is friendly to read; however, the findings do not appear to be saying anything new, and it had potential to be much richer.

2. The paper portrays it as easy to work with these clients and this may not be the case.

3. The paper is brave and ploughs a furrow, inviting others to come on board and debate and discuss, and therefore is valuable.

References

Babiker, I. E. and Thorne, P. (1993) Do psychiatric patients know what is good for them? *Journal of the Royal Sociaty of Medicine*, **86**, 28–30.

Beech, P. and Norman, I. J. (1995) Patients' perceptions of the quality of psychiatric nurisng care: findings from a small-scale descriptive study. *Journal of Clinical Nursing*, **4**, 117–23.

Benner, P. (1984) *From Novice to Expert: Excellence and Power in Clinical Nursing Practice*. Addison-Wesley, Menlo Park, CA.

Benner, P. and Wrubel, J. (1989) *The Primacy of Caring: Stress and Coping in Health and Illness*. Addison-Wesley, Menlo Park, CA.

Burnard, P. and Chapman, C. (2003) *Professional and Ethical Issues in Nursing*, 3rd edn. Baillière Tindall, Edinburgh.

Campbell, P. (1998) Listening to clients. In: *Psychiatric Nursing: Ethical Strife* (eds. P. Barker and B. Davidson), pp. 237–48. Arnold, London.

Cormack, D. (1983) *Psychiatric Nursing Described*. Churchill Livingstone, Edinburgh.

Denzin, N. K. and Lincoln, Y. S. (1994) Entering the field of qualitative research. In: *A Handbook of Qualitative Research* (eds. N. K. Denzin and Y. S. Lincoln), pp. 1–17. Sage, California.

Department of Health (1994) *Working in Partnership: a Collaborative Approach to Care. Report of the Mental Health Nursing Review Team.* HMSO, London.

Duffy, D. and Lee, R. (1998) Mental health nursing today: ideal and reality. *Mental Health Practice,* 1(8), 14–16.

Elbeck, M. and Fecteau, G. (1990) Improving the validity of measures of patient satisfaction with psychiatric care and treatment. *Hospital and Community Psychiatry,* 41(9), 998–1001.

Elzinga, R. H. and Barlow, J. (1991) Patient satisfaction among the residentail population of a psychiatric hospital. *International Journal of Social Psychiatry,* 37(1), 24–34.

Gallop, R. (1997) Caring about the client: the role of gender, empathy and power in the therapeutic process. In: *The Mental Health Nurse: Views of Practice and Education* (eds. S. Tilley), pp. 28–42. Blackwell Science, London.

Heidegger, M. (1962) *Being and Time.* Harper & Row, New York.

Hill, B. and Michael, S. (1996) The human factor. *Journal of Psychiatric and Mental Health Nursing,* 3, 245–8.

Lincoln, Y. S. and Guba, E. G. (1985) *Naturalistic Inquiry.* Sage, London.

Lipson, J. (1994) The use of self in ethnographic research. In: *Qualitative Nursing Research: a Contemporary Dialogue* (ed. J. M. Morse), pp. 73–89. Sage, London.

Lovell, K. (1995) User satisfaction with in-patient mental health services. *Journal of Psychiatric and Mental Health Nursing,* 2, 143–50.

McHale, J. and Gallagher, A. (2003) *Nursing and Human Rights.* Butterworth-Heinemann, London.

McIver, S. (1991a) *An Introduction to Obtaining the Views of Users of Health Services.* King's Fund Centre, London.

McIver, S. (1991b) *Obtaining the Views of Users of Mental Health Services.* King's Fund Centre, London.

Melia, K. M. (1982) 'Tell it as it is' – qualitative methodology and nursing research: understanding the student nurse's world. *Journal of Advanced Nursing,* 7, 327–35.

Mental Health Foundation (2000) *Strategies for Living.* Mental Health Foundation, London.

MIND (1986) *Finding Our Own Solutions: Women's Experiences of Mental Health Care.* National Association for Mental Health, London.

Morse, J. M. (1991) Strategies for sampling. In: *Qualitative Nursing Research: a Contemporary Dialogue* (ed. J. M. Morse), pp. 126–45. Sage, London.

Patton, M. Q. (1990) *Qualitative Evaluation and Research Methods,* 2nd edn. Sage, London.

Pickett, S. A., Lyons, J. S., Polonus, T., Seymour, T. and Miller, S. I. (1993) Factors predicting satisfaction with managed mental health care. *Psychiatric Services,* 46(7), 722–3.

Repper, J., Ford, R. and Cooke, A. (1994) How can nurses build trusting relationships with people who have severe and long-term mental health problems? Experiences of case managers and their clients. *Journal of Advanced Nursing,* 19, 1096–104.

Sheppard, M. (1993) Client satisfaction, extended intervention and interpersonal skills in community mental health. *Journal of Advanced Nursing,* 18, 246–59.

Stephenson, C., Wilson, S. and Gladman, J. R. F. (1995) Patient and carer satisfaction in geriatric day hospitals. *Disability and Rehabilitation,* 17(5), 252–5.

Streubert, H. J. and Carpenter, D. R. (1999) *Qualitative Research in Nursing: Advancing the Humanistic Imperative.* Lippincott, Philadelphia.

Towell, D. (1975) *Understanding Psychiatric Nursing,* RCN London.

Van Manen, M. (1997) *Researching Lived Experience: Human Science for Action Sensitive Pedagogy.* State University of New York Press, New York.

Walters, A. J. (1995) The phenomenological movement: implications for nursing research. *Journal of Advanced Nursing,* 22, 791–9.

Example 14: The NPNR National Journal Club: review of the 5th meeting

The paper reviewed was Rogers, T. S. and Kashima, Y. (1998) Nurses' responses to people with schizophrenia. *Journal of Advanced Nursing*, **27**, 195–203.

Abstract/overview

This paper reports on a study that investigated differences between general nurses, P/MH nurses and lay people. It attempted to identify differences between their personal standards concerning how they should respond, and beliefs about how they actually would respond to people with schizophrenia. Evidence of these differences was examined in each of three domains: thinking, feeling and behaving. Significant differences were identified between the response types and between the different response domains. Significant interaction effects were also identified based on participants' professional status in nursing. The authors argue that their results support Devine's (1989) theory concerning the automatic activation of stereotypes and their controlled inhibition in favour of different personal beliefs. The authors additionally argue that professional socialisation in psychiatric nursing facilitates this process with relation to people with schizophrenia.

Title

Feedback comments indicated that members felt the title was somewhat misleading. The study contained an examination of three groups of people, including lay people. However, the title makes no reference to the examination of lay people's responses.

Abstract

Members expressed that the abstract introduced the focus of the study, gave a brief outline of the method and identified the major findings of the report.

Introduction

It was felt that the introduction included the appropriate background to the study and a rationale for undertaking it.

Background literature

Members stated that they felt that the background literature section was well written, comprehensive, easy to read and thorough. It offered a balanced argument and drew upon a wide range of appropriate literature. Additional comments stated that it might be argued that within the list of terms regarded as positive, in addition to the term 'sensitive', that the stereotypical traits 'strong, convincing, active and mysterious' could be construed as positive evaluative statements (Facchia *et al.*, 1976).

The hypothesis

It is reasonable to say that the response regarding the paper's hypotheses was mixed, although there was a range of criticism. Comments ranged from a feeling that the first two hypotheses led to a confirmation of the obvious, and therefore led to members wondering 'what would this confirmation add to the knowledge base?'. Additionally, members stated that they felt the third hypothesis could be regarded as somewhat obsolete since the introduction of Project 2000 nurse training programmes and the introduction of Common Foundation programmes. An alternative view was expressed that asserted that differences in emphasis, philosophical underpinning, attitude, knowledge and skills base still exist between P/MH and general nurses. Consequently, research into this issue and a hypothesis of this nature might be regarded as entirely appropriate.

Method

Members stated that they felt that the method was appropriate to the study design and stated research questions; however, it still raised some questions. The first question centred around why the pilot study did not sample the same population as the main study. According to Polit and Hungler (1997), the purpose of a pilot study is to carry out a small scale version or trial run of the major study in order to obtain information for improving the project or assessing its feasibility. Other authors (for example, Bond, 1991; Peat, 2002; Hicks, 2004) make similar remarks and indicate that if a pilot study is carried out on a small number of subjects, it may help to answer a number of questions, including whether or not the subjects can understand what is being asked of them. Considering that this questionnaire would need to be completed by lay people, it would appear to have been wise to screen it for nursing jargon and the excessive use of medical terminology. Consequently, members wondered what value would be obtained by conducting the pilot study on a group of 15 nurse academics?[1]

Another question concerned the methods of data collection, in particular encouraging the respondents to complete the questionnaires in small groups. Members expressed concern that such a method of data collection could have influenced the results due to peer pressure, and wondered why the participants were not encouraged to complete the questionnaires on their own. While the authors may have had a plausible rationale for such a method, this was not highlighted in the paper. A further

---

1 In addition to the point made above, Peat (2002) purports that the following processes can be evaluated by means of a pilot study: the quality of the data collection forms and the accuracy of the instruments; the practicalities of conducting the study; the success of recruitment approaches; the feasibility of subject compliance with tests; and estimates for use in sample size calculations.

question related to the collection of the data for the section of the study concerned with 'should *vs*. would' responses to people with schizophrenia. It was argued that the design is weakened by the fact that what respondents 'would do' had to be taken on trust. The authors do point out that there was no evidence of the respondents trying to portray themselves in the most favourable light possible, but these criticisms could have been prevented by the inclusion of an observation element, perhaps using simulators (Faulkner 1994). Simulated or role-played events could have been created and the responses to these events observed.

Sample

Members raised concerns regarding the nature of the sample composition. The authors described the average age of the respondents for each of the three groups sampled and the ratio of male/female. The average age of the psychiatric nurses was five years older than the remainder of the sample. This produced a situation where the psychiatric nurses had significantly more clinical experience than their general colleagues. There was a further difference between the number of males in the different sample groups. Consequently it could be argued that the authors were not comparing like with like (Parahoo, 1997; Polit *et al.*, 2001). Any differences that exist in responses from the different groups could then be attributed to any of the variables and not necessarily the dependent variable. It should be noted that the authors do make some reference to the age difference between the groups and how this could affect the results. However, they do not acknowledge the variation in clinical experience or the proportion of males to females as possible explanations for the differences in response to the questionnaire.

Ethical considerations

The authors stated that ethical approval had been obtained before the study commenced; however, some of the members stated that they would have liked to have seen some more detail regarding ethical approval. For example, all research involving human subjects is carried out at some cost to the participants. While this cost may be difficult to identify or may appear trivial, humans as subjects need and deserve appropriate respect and protection (McHale and Gallagher, 2003; Burnard and Chapman, 2003).

Data analysis

Members' feedback indicated that they felt the data analysis section lacked detail. The paper is somewhat imprecise with regard to the research design, in that it appears to be using a phenomenological method, yet it does not make this clear. However, the major criticism of this section was the lack of a comprehensive explanation of how the themes were induced. Members wanted to see how the researchers had moved from labels (initial categorisation) to condensing these into 'main problem areas' to the central themes. Additionally, it would have been useful to see how the themes/categorisations interrelated with one another.

Results

The range of responses regarding the results was mixed. Some members reported that they felt it included the appropriate analysis for the data collected (Burnard and Morrison, 1990), contained a high number of charts, tables and graphs and used a substantial amount of research terminology. Consequently, members described this section as well written and informative. However, other members felt that the use of terminology and jargon could be regarded as excessive. Comments included concerns regarding how many nurses would be discouraged from reading and assimilating the paper due to the use of terminology. These concerns have been expressed by several authors, e.g. Hunt (1981), Miller (1985), and Lobiondo-Wood and Haber (1986), and more recently in related disciplines such as occupational therapy (Creek, 2006). The variation of opinion expressed by the members regarding this issue highlights something of a dichotomy facing authors of research reports. It is likely that such authors wish to reach as many people as possible with their research, as their findings thus have an increased chance of affecting thinking and/or practice. Therefore they may wish to use a minimum of terminology. At the same time they may feel the need to appear knowledgeable and credible to their academic peers. Consequently, questions and dilemmas exist for authors concerning the issue of how much terminology is excessive.

Discussion, conclusions and recommendations

Members stated that factors appeared to be omitted from the discussion. They pointed out that they had witnessed the phenomenon of negative stereotypes of mentally ill people present in general nurses being replaced by more positive views as a result of spending time with clients while on clinical placement, thus supporting the findings of the authors. However, the members described how these positive views were only temporary in that once the general nursing students became re-socialised into their peer group and general nursing clinical placements, the positive views were undermined and they once more adopted the more negative stereotypes. Therefore it appears to be possible that a change in people's stereotypes of individuals with mental health problems may be related to the length of time of exposure to such people or the intensity of the exposure. The article highlighted some interesting lines of inquiry for possible future research and recognised some of the study's limitations.

Final comments: What meaning does this have for psychiatric and mental health nurses?

The article pointed out differences between general nurses and P/MH nurses in their responses to people with schizophrenia. Some members argued that this was a confirmation of the obvious, namely that graded exposure to the stereotyped target group decreases negative responses in the thinking and feeling domain (Nolan, 1993). Other members felt that these findings add to the argument that there are differences in emphasis, philosophical underpinning, attitudes, knowledge and skills between general and P/MH nurses. Recent attempts to explicate these differences (Cutcliffe and McKenna, 2000a,b) included the identification of eight alleged elements of the uniqueness of P/MH nurses. These included the ability to work in ordinary ways with extra-ordinary people; the human component of P/MH nursing, best seen as the craft of nursing; forming and maintaining relationships founded on empathy; and the endeavours to form partnerships with clients and work in collaboration with clients.

The findings of the reviewed study perhaps support these elements, in that in order to form empathic relationships, establish partnerships and work in ordinary ways with extra-ordinary people, the P/MH has first to come to terms with his/her own internal prejudices and agendas (Cutcliffe, 1995). As Benner and Wrubel (1989, p. 12) state:

> The nurse has in some sense personally come to terms with the reality of the illness and is able to convey acceptance and understanding to the patient.

Skilled P/MH nurses then can be regarded as people who can acknowledge their personal prejudices, thoughts and feelings, and who can hold such perceptions in abeyance, allowing them to be challenged and re-framed into more positive perceptions, enough to be able to work with people who provoke negative stereotypes.

Table 10.2 Key points arising from review No. 5.

1. The paper adds to the debate surrounding the issue of the differences in emphasis between psychiatric/mental health nurses and general nurses, and perhaps indicates a component of the alleged uniqueness of psychiatric/mental health nurses that Nolan (1993) alluded to.

2. The paper confirms the continuing presence and influence of negative stereotypes of people who suffer from mental health problems and provides useful evidence on one method to counteract such stereotypes.

3. Perhaps the extent of the terminology or jargon included in the text may distance some potential readers, thus minimising the potential impact of the article.

References

Benner, P. and Wrubel, J. (1989) *The Primacy of Caring: Stress and Coping in Health and Wellness.* Addison-Wesley, New York.

Bond, S. (1991) Preparing a research proposal. In: *The Research Process in Nursing*, 2nd edn (ed. D. Cormack). Blackwell Science, London.

Burnard, P. and Chapman, C. (2003) *Professional and Ethical Issues in Nursing*, 3rd edn. Baillière Tindall, Edinburgh.

Creek, J. (2006) Finding the right words: the significance of professional terminology. *International Journal of Therapy and Rehabilitation*, **13**(1), 6.

Cutcliffe, J. R. (1995) How do nurses inspire and instil hope in terminally ill HIV people? *Journal of Advanced Nursing*, **22**, 888–95.

Cutcliffe, J. R. and McKenna, H. P. (2000a) Generic nurses: the nemesis of psychiatric/mental health nursing? Part One. *Mental Health Practice*, **3**(9), 10–14.

Cutcliffe, J. R. and McKenna, H. P. (2000b) Generic nurses: the nemesis of psychiatric/mental health nursing? Part Two. *Mental Health Practice*, **3**(10), 20–3.

Devine, P. G. (1989) Stereotypes and prejudices: their automatic and controlled components. *Journal of Personal Social Psychology*, **55**(1), 5–18.

Facchia, J., Canale, D., Cambria, E., Ruest, E. and Sheppard, C. (1976) Public views of ex-mental patients: a note on perceived dangerousness and unpredictability. *Psychological Reports*, **38**(2), 495–8.

Faulkner, A. (1994) Using simulators to aid the teaching of communication skills in cancer and palliative care. *Patient Education and Counselling*, **23**, 125–9.

Hicks, C. (2004) *Research Methods for Clinical Therapists: Applied Project Design and Analysis*. Churchill Livingstone, Edinburgh.

Hunt, J. (1981) The process of translating research findings into practice. *Journal of Advanced Nursing*, **12**, 101–10.

LoBiondo-Wood, G. and Haber, J. (1986) *Nursing Research, Critical Appraisal and Utilisation*. C. V. Mosby, Toronto.

Nolan, P. (1993) *A History of Mental Health Nursing*. Chapman & Hall, London.

Miller, A. (1985) The relationship between nursing theory and nursing practice. *Journal of Advanced Nursing*, **10**, 417–24.

Parahoo, K. (1997) *Nursing Research: Principles, Process and Issues*. Macmillan Press, London.

Peat, J. (2002) *Health Science Research: A Handbook of Quantitative Methods*. Sage, London.

Polit, D. F. and Hungler, B. P. (1997) *Essentials of Nursing Research: Methods, Appraisal and Utilisation*, 4th edn. Lippincott, Philadelphia.

Polit, D. F., Beck, C. T. and Hungler, B. P. (2001) *Essentials of Nursing Research: Methods, Appraisal and Utilization*, 5th edn. Lippincott, Philadelphia.

CHAPTER 11

The third stage of the NPNR Journal Club development: gaining confidence in the approach

Example 15: The NPNR National Journal Club: review from the 6th meeting

The paper reviewed was Waite, A., Carson, J., Cullen, D., Oliver, N., Holloway, F. and Missenden, K. (1997) Case management: a week in the life of a clinical case management team. *Journal of Psychiatric and Mental Health Nursing*, **4**, 285–94.

Abstract/overview

This paper reports on a study that attempted to describe the work of a clinical case management core team. The researchers gathered information through non-participant observation and went on to produce transcripts which were subsequently examined. From these transcripts the authors produced seven categories of activity which were felt to encompass the range of activities practised by the team: planned client contact; unplanned client contact; family/carer contact; liaison; administration; team information sharing and supervision; and training and personal development. The authors also calculated the amount of time engaged in these activities and their results were discussed in reference to Kanter's components and principles of clinical case management.

Title

Feedback comments indicated that members felt the title identified the focus of the research study, but perhaps could have been improved by including an indication of the methodology used.

Abstract

Members felt that the abstract introduced the focus of the study, gave a brief outline of the method and identified the major findings of the report.

Introduction

Some members stated that the introduction included an appropriate background to the study, in that the authors identify problems with case management, particularly in the way researchers have rarely given adequate descriptions of the precise nature of the service they are investigating. However, some concerns were expressed concerning the way the introduction appears to merge with a review of selected literature and consequently they struggled to easily identify the current level of knowledge or understanding of this phenomenon. This has particular implications for the selection of an appropriate methodology (see below). Other members reported further confusion arising from the introduction. The introduction indicates that the general aims/principles and the core functions of case management have been identified. It then goes on to say that few studies provide adequate descriptions. Therefore, since the authors have cited these studies, a logical question is: how do these previous studies describe clinical case management and what do they say it is? Would it not have been appropriate to include and then critique such definitions if they exist?

The confusion is perhaps cleared up somewhat in the next section of the paper, where the authors highlight the absence of any literature that details the actual process of clinical case management. Therefore, some members felt it might have been more appropriate to use this as the justification for the study as such arguments appear to be cogent and robust.

Method

Members stated that they felt there were several possible flaws with the method and research design. First was the issue of precision and clarity. The paper under review appears to have an absence of precision and clarity. All the readers are told is that it used a qualitative method (p. 289). Stern (1994) submitted that although there may be similarities in all interpretative methods, the frameworks underlying the methods differ. Baker *et al.* (1992) constructed similar arguments, and furthermore they reasoned that failure to explicate qualitative methodologies is resulting in a body of nursing research that is mislabelled. Similarly, Morse (1991, p. 15) warned of this mixing of methods and stressed that:

> the product is not good science; the product is a sloppy mishmash.

Thus, by paying attention to the resolution or precision of qualitative research methodology the researcher is endeavouring to ensure rigour (Baker *et al.*, 1992). Such rigorous studies should 'stand up' better to critique by enabling the reader to examine whether or not the chosen methodology was appropriate to the nature of the research study. Furthermore, some members questioned whether or not it was accurate to describe this paper as a qualitative study, since the handling and presentation of the data provided little insight into the subjective worlds of the participants. This apparent confusion regarding the methodology may be further evidenced by the authors' use of the terms *reliability* and *validity*, and perhaps the presence and influence of Kanter's theory in the minds of the researcher during data collection and analysis.

In considering these arguments, there is a need to examine the philosophical underpinnings of quantitative research approaches. A researcher who adopts a quantitative approach to the collection of data is viewing the world through a particular type of lens. The view suggests that the world can be explained and understood in terms of universal laws and objective truths (McKenna, 1997). Its positivist and empiricist underpinnings suggest that there is only one reality, and consequently a measure of the accuracy of this reality is its validity.

However, the qualitative researcher views the world through a very different lens. Key authorities on qualitative research point out that it is inappropriate to attempt to apply positivistic and empiricist views of the world to qualitative research (Benner and Wrubel, 1989; Morse, 1991; Denzin and Lincoln, 1994; Cutcliffe and McKenna 1999, 2002; Angen, 2000; Rolfe, 2006). Qualitative research is based upon the belief that there is no one singular universal truth, the social world is multi-faceted, it is an outcome of the interaction of human agents, a world that has no unequivocal reality (Ashworth, 1997). It is concerned with describing, interpreting and understanding the meaning that people attribute to their existence and to their world.

Consequently, qualitative research findings should be tested for credibility or accuracy using terms and criteria that have been developed exclusively for this very approach (Hammersley, 1992; Cutcliffe and McKenna, 1999, 2002; Angen, 2000; Rolfe, 2006). Leininger (1994) makes this point most clearly when she states:

> we must develop and use criteria that fit the qualitative paradigm, rather than use quantitative criteria for qualitative studies. It is awkward and inappropriate to re-language quantitative terms.

Some members wondered if the presence and potential influence of Kanter's theory moved the study away from being an inductive study and moved it toward a deductive study. The existence of such an existing theory raises questions about the research design. According to Morse and Field (1995, p. 8):

> the researcher should selectively and appropriately choose a research approach according to the nature of the problem and what is known about the phenomenon to be studied.

Therefore, if a theory already exists that provides definitions, principles and components of clinical case management, was it appropriate to attempt to use a qualitative method? Given Morse and Field's (1995) argument, maybe there would have been more merit in testing Kanter's theory (a deductive study). Additionally, in some ways that appears to be what the authors have done. Members identified further problems pertaining to the method section. Some wondered what constituted an 'activity' for the purposes of this study and suggested that the authors could have included a definition. Furthermore, how was the information recorded? What endeavours did the authors make to minimise the impact of the Hawthorne Effect (Polit and Hungler, 1997; Polit et al., 2001; Hicks, 2004)?

Data analysis

A criticism raised by the members was the lack of a comprehensive explanation of how the themes were induced. Members wanted to see how the researchers had moved from labels (initial categorisation) to condensing these into 'main problem areas' to the central themes. Also, it would have been useful to see how the themes/categorisations interrelated with one another. Members wondered if this was further evidence of the lack of precision or clarity evident in this paper.

Ethical considerations

The absence of any ethical considerations or details regarding ethical approval was felt to be an oversight (Lipson, 1994). The paper contained no mention of ethical considerations. All research involving human subjects is carried out at some cost to the participants. While this cost may be difficult to identify or may appear trivial, the humans as subjects need and deserve appropriate respect and protection (Royal College of Nursing, 1998; McHale and Gallagher, 2003; Burnard and Chapman, 2003).

Results

It is reasonable to say that the range of responses regarding the results section was mixed. Some members reported certain discrepancies in the results. For example, the pie chart indicates a figure of 35% for the total time that case managers devoted to client contact. Yet the discussion (p. 292) refers to 38% and not 35% (p. 293). Furthermore, page 292 states that team information sharing and staff support/development account for 31% of the case managers' time. However, adding these two figures together from the pie chart figures adds up to 29%.

Other comments indicated the usefulness of the examples (from work outside of the observed week) used to add to the richness of the understanding. It was noted that planned client contact was the only category that has such examples to support the findings and members wondered why this was the case. Was it that no data was available? Arguably, the theory would be richer for such examples (Cassell, 2004).

Discussion, conclusions and recommendations

Opinions were divided regarding this section. The discussion raises some important issues, particularly those pertaining to smaller caseloads and recognising the need to fulfil important additional tasks. Also, comments regarding the need for ongoing clinical supervision were met with overwhelming support from the members. This argument continues to be raised in the literature (Butterworth and Faugier, 1992; Bond and Holland, 1998). The findings from this paper further add to the qualitative evidence supporting the widespread uptake and use of clinical supervision. Concerns were raised about how the paper appears to move into comparing contact numbers, and thus towards a quantitative methodology. Yet such an endeavour falls outside of the stated aim of the paper and added to the overall positivistic 'flavour' of the paper.

Members expressed some concern regarding the use of 'sweeping generalisations' in the discussion, such as 'research shows that working in the community is more stressful than working in hospital settings'. Given that stress is such a personal and individualised reaction (Rawlins et al., 1993; Myers, 1998), it is at best unwise to make such claims. Members did not doubt the accuracy of such findings, but felt that it would have been more appropriate to cite the results in more detail.

Final comments: what meaning does this have for psychiatric and mental health nurses?

What this paper does do is add to the debate concerning the nature of P/MH nursing practice. According to Duffy and Lee (1998), Hopton (1997) and Cutcliffe and McKenna (2000a,b), P/MH nurses in the United Kingdom (UK) find themselves in a position of uncertainty and subsequently P/MH nursing is deeply immersed in a crisis of legitimacy. Whether or not P/MH nurses should lose their specialist status and become generic nurses is based on the argument that there is compelling evidence to support the introduction of multi-skilling and cross-training (HMSU, 1996). Yet opponents of such a position maintain that there is something crucial and unique in P/MH nursing which is distinct and worth preserving (Nolan, 1993). Nonetheless, the literature is at best unclear regarding the precise nature of this uniqueness. Cutcliffe and McKenna (2000a) assert that this lack of precision is one of the problems and if P/MH nurses are unable to articulate what their contribution is and what the nature of this uniqueness is, then arguably it is more difficult to defend this distinctiveness.

Consequently the paper reviewed can be seen to be attempting to identify elements of this uniqueness, since a key element of this process is describing what these nurses do. However, perhaps the problems with the method compromise the credibility or validity of this theory. Therefore further qualitative inquiry is needed to identify the nature of the alleged uniqueness of P/MH nurses.

References

Angen, M. J. (2000) Evaluating interpretive inquiry: reviewing the validity debate and opening the dialogue. *Qualitative Health Research*, **10**(3), 378–95.

Ashworth, P. D. (1997) The variety of qualitative research: non-positivist approaches. *Nurse Education Today*, **17**, 219–24.

Table 11.1 Key points arising from review No. 6.

1. The paper appears to have some confusion regarding the methodology, evidenced by the authors' inappropriate use of the terms *reliability* and *validity*, and perhaps the presence and influence of Kanter's theory in the minds of the researchers during data collection and analysis. Members questioned whether or not it was accurate to describe this paper as a qualitative study, since the handling and presentation of the data provided little insight into the subjective worlds of the participants.

2. The paper can be seen to be furnishing the argument that psychiatric/ mental health nurses provide a unique contribution, since a key element of this process is describing what these nurses do.

3. The paper might have been served by attention to issues of methodological precision. Such mindfulness and the resulting methodological rigour is likely to increase the overall quality of the inquiry and enhance the credibility of the findings.

Baker, C., Wuest, J. and Stern, P. N. (1992) Method slurring: the grounded theory/phenomenology example. *Journal of Advanced Nursing*, **17**, 1355–60.

Benner, P. and Wrubel, J. (1989) *The Primacy of Caring: Stress and Coping in Health and Illness*. Addison-Wesley, New York.

Bond, M. and Holland, S. (1998) *Skills of Clinical Supervision for Nurses*. Open University Press, Oxford.

Burnard, P. and Chapman, C. (2003) *Professional and Ethical Issues in Nursing*, 3rd edn. Baillière Tindall, Edinburgh.

Butterworth, T. and Faugier, J. (1992) Supervision for life. In: *Clinical Supervision and Mentorship in Nursing* (eds. T. Butterworth and J. Faugier), pp. 230–40. Chapman & Hall, London.

Cassell, C. (2004) *Essential Guide to Qualitative Methods in Organizational Research*. Sage, London.

Cutcliffe, J. R. and McKenna, H. P. (1999) Establishing the credibility of qualitative research findings: the plot thickens. *Journal of Advanced Nursing*, **30**(2), 374–80.

Cutcliffe, J. R. and McKenna, H. P. (2000a) Generic nurses: the nemesis of psychiatric/mental health nursing? Part One. *Mental Health Practice*, **3**(9), 10–14.

Cutcliffe, J. R. and McKenna, H. P. (2000b) Generic nurses: the nemesis of psychiatric/mental health nursing? Part Two. *Mental Health Practice*, **3**(4), 20–3.

Cutcliffe, J. R. and McKenna, H. P. (2002) When do we know that we know? Considering the truth of research findings and the craft of qualitative research. *International Journal of Nursing Studies*, **39**(6), 611–18.

Denzin, N. and Lincoln, Y. S. (1994) Introduction: entering the field of qualitative enquiry. In: *Handbook of Qualitative Research* (eds. N. Denzin and Y. S. Lincoln). Sage, London.

Duffy, D. and Lee, R. (1998) Mental health nursing today: ideal and reality. *Mental Health Practice*, **1**(8), 14–16.

Hammersley, M. (1992) *What's Wrong with Ethnography?* Routledge, London.

Hicks, C. (2004) *Research Methods for Clinical Therapists: Applied Project Design and Analysis*, 4th edn. Churchill Livingstone, Edinburgh.

HMSU – University of Manchester (1996) *The Future Healthcare Workforce: the Steering Group Report*. Health Services Management Group, Manchester.

Hopton, J. (1997) Towards a critical theory of mental health nursing. *Journal of Advanced Nursing*, **25**, 492–500.

Leininger, M. (1994) Evaluation criteria and critique of qualitative research studies. In: *Critical Issues in Qualitative Research Methods* (ed. J. M. Morse). Sage, Thousand Oaks.

Lipson, J. (1994) The use of self in ethnographic research. In: *Qualitative Nursing Research: a Contemporary Dialogue* (ed J. M. Morse), pp. 73–89. Sage, London.

McHale, J. and Gallagher, A. (2003) *Nursing and Human Rights*. Butterworth-Heinemann, London.

McKenna, H. P. (1997) *Nursing Theories and Models*. Routledge, London.

Morse, J. M. (1991) Qualitative nursing research: a free for all. In: *Qualitative Nursing Research: a Contemporary Dialogue* (ed. J. M. Morse), pp. 14–22. Sage, London.

Morse, J. M. and Field, P. A. (1995) *Qualitative Research Methods for Health Professionals*. 2nd edn. Sage, London.

Myers, D. G. (1998) *Psychology*, 5th edn. Worth, New York.

Nolan, P. (1993) *A History of Mental Health Nursing*. Chapman & Hall, London.

Polit, D. F. and Hungler, B. P. (1993) *Essentials of Nursing Research: Methods, Appraisal and Utilization*, 3rd edn. Lippincott, Philadelphia.

Polit, D. F., Beck, C. T. and Hungler, B. P. (2001) *Essentials of Nursing Research: Methods, Appraisal and Utilization*, 5th edn. Lippincott, Philadelphia.

Rawlins, R. P., Williams, S. R. and Beck, C. K. (1993) *Mental Health Psychiatric Nursing: a Holistic Life-Cycle Approach*. C. V. Mosby, St Louis.

Royal College of Nursing (1998) *Research Ethics: Guidelines for Nurses Involved in Research Or Any Investigative Project Involving Human Subjects*. Royal College of Nursing, London.

Rolfe, G. (2006) Judgments without rules: towards a postmodern ironist concept of research validity. *Nursing Inquiry*, **13**, 7–15.

Stern, P. N. (1994) Eroding grounded theory. In: *Critical Issues in Qualitative Research Methods* (ed. J. M. Morse), pp. 210–23. Sage, London.

Streubert, H. J. and Carpenter, D. R. (1999) *Qualitative Research in Nursing: Advancing the Humanistic Imperative*. Lippincott, London.

Example 14: The NPNR National Journal Club: review from the 7th meeting

The paper reviewed was Gass, J. P. (1998) The knowledge and attitudes of mental health nurses to electro-convulsive therapy. *Journal of Advanced Nursing*, **27**, 83–90.

Abstract/overview

This paper reports on a study that attempted to elicit the knowledge and attitudes of P/MH nurses about electro-convulsive therapy (ECT). One hundred and sixty seven questionnaires containing attitude/knowledge scales were returned from the 345 sent out. The author discovered limitations in the reliability of the instrument and thus reliable measures of the respondents' knowledge of ECT were not obtained. The author's findings indicated correlations with higher levels of knowledge and (a) length of experience and (b) area of clinical practice. He also noted significant variations in knowledge of cognitive side effects. The author concludes that nurses' knowledge of ECT requires improvement in many cases and that this has implications for nurse education.

Title

Feedback comments from the members regarding the title were mixed, with some saying that the title clearly identified the focus of the research, while others felt that the title could have indicated something of the research approach, the methodology or the design.

Abstract

Members expressed that given the limited space the abstract managed to convey the core of what the paper was about. However, perhaps the author could have included some detail about the sample, and it said nothing about the context within which the study took place.

Introduction

Some members stated that the introduction was concise and to the point, whereas others felt that again it provided no context as to why the research was undertaken. It is possible that this section of the text would have been strengthened by including some justification for the study. Members were left wondering whether the study was conducted in response to a national issue or agenda, as a result of some increasing trend in the use of ECT, or as a result of the author's particular interest in this subject.

Literature review

If the bulk of the comments for the preceding sections were positive, it is reasonable to say that the members expressed more criticism of the literature review. In this section the author suggests that ECT can be regarded as a form of punishment. While few would disagree that this can be the case, ECT is clearly not the only 'medical' or even nursing treatment/intervention that can be regarded in this way; e.g. the administration of tranquilising medication (particularly after a violent incident), the use of seclusion rooms, and indeed 'punishment therapy' (Masson, 1992).

Most of the literature focuses on papers that discuss the advantages and disadvantages of ECT. It is only in the last two paragraphs that papers describing similar studies are mentioned. This left members wondering whether these are the only studies of this kind. Thus concerns were expressed regarding the balance of the literature and whether this was a comprehensive review or important papers had been omitted – for example Dr Liam Clarke's (1995) paper 'Psychiatric nursing and ECT'. There was, notably, no mention of the complexities associated with attitudinal measurement, little on nurses and nothing much on conscientious objection to health care interventions. The literature review made no mention of who receives ECT, and this could be particularly relevant as P/MH nurses' attitudes towards ECT may well be dissimilar for different 'conditions' or 'illnesses'.

Method

The members stated that they felt there were several flaws with the method. The author selected a convenience sample and while this may have been appropriate, he could have explored the advantages and disadvantages of using such a sample. Additionally, a rationale for choosing this sampling strategy may have been beneficial. The author used a data collection tool which had been used in a previous study. However, the author acknowledges that this tool produced low reliability scores which left the members wondering, given that this tool had already been identified as having a low reliability, then why choose this tool and not another one? Perhaps the choice of this tool is linked to an incomplete or limited literature review, in that this may have been the only tool that was uncovered in the literature.

Further methodological difficulties were evident in the adoption of a tool designed to measure attitudes in the USA. Attitudes are influenced by the pervading culture and sub-cultures (Hammersley, 1992; Stanfield, 1994; Cassell, 2004) and it is thus unlikely that nurses in the USA have the same culture to nurses in Britain. Members expressed that insufficient detail was provided on the method used and the rationale for choosing this method. It may have been worthwhile for the author to have explored alternative scoring systems, for example using questions with visual analogue scales, which have particular value in measuring subjective experiences and this would have been more in keeping with measuring attitudes (Polit and Hungler, 1997; Peat, 2002; Hicks, 2004).

Since the author's sample was comprised entirely from two trusts, it is conceivable that the nurses' attitudes could well have been influenced by another local ECT policy that existed and it might have been useful to see an overview of such policies (if they existed). In terms of the low response rate the author acknowledges this, and it should be noted that he made efforts to increase the response rate with the use of a follow-up letter. However, in terms of the research design, members questioned the logic in sending out questionnaires at Christmas time (although this probably coincided with the author's dissertation schedule). Maybe the author's pilot study could have identified certain clinical areas that would be unlikely to provide a comprehensive response to such questionnaires, such as those areas who do not invest heavily in ETC. Yet no breakdown of response rate to the pilot study according to clinical area is included.

A further problem identified with the method was that respondents were instructed to choose between ECT, pharmacological intervention and psychotherapy. Yet many of the members declared that more often than not these treatments are concomitant, and therefore deciding between them is not a reflection of practice.

Ethical considerations

The absence of any ethical considerations or details regarding ethical approval was felt to be an oversight (Lipson, 1994; Burnard and Chapman, 2003). The paper contained no mention of ethical considerations. All research involving human subjects is carried out at some cost to the participants. While this cost may be difficult to identify or may appear trivial, the humans as subjects need and deserve appropriate respect and protection (Royal College of Nursing, 1998; McHale and Gallagher, 2003).

Findings

It is reasonable to say that the members raised several criticisms regarding the findings section. The demographic details of the sample were described in this section, which only served to confuse matters. If the author included these details in order to enable a repeat of his study in the future, members felt that it would have been more appropriate to include the details of the sample under a separate sub-title. If the author included these details in order to carry out some analysis, for example, to look for correlations between the sex of the respondents and their knowledge/attitudes, then it would be entirely appropriate to include the details in this section. Yet no such correlations are examined, which left some of the members wondering about inattentive construction of questionnaires.

Two surprising, and possibly noteworthy, observations are that no Project 2000 (P2K) students were included in the sample, and secondly, that more than half the sample were aged 40 years or over. Was it that the study was completed before the advent of P2K or was there some other unstated reason for this omission? A significant criticism was that, contrary to the author's over-zealous attention to the results, no really significant differences between the groups of nurses responding existed. The mean differences in knowledge scores between 'elderly care' nurses and 'acute care' nurses differed very little. Yet the discussion made an awful lot of not very much. Perhaps this does raise an interesting point about when do differences become significant and who decides? The author's comment on p. 86 regarding 'elderly care' nurses having their knowledge based more exclusively on biomedical literature was felt to be inappropriate and inaccurate, especially when one considers Kitwood and Benson's (1995) work, Nolan *et al*.'s (1997) research and many 'elderly care' nurses' arguments that they provide holistic, multi-dimensional care rather than bio-medically orientated, physical care (Ross, 1997; Pulsford, 1997).

The relatively small differences in knowledge (less than 1.5) are raised as an issue by the author and he explains these differences in part as a result of the degree of experience. He also states that the knowledge did not vary according to the nurses' qualifications. Thus, it is unlikely that the education/training is responsible for any differences in knowledge. Yet the author suggests that such differences in knowledge could be addressed in nurse education, which is somewhat illogical.

The author also argues that exposure to ECT is not associated with differences in knowledge of ECT, yet on p. 87 he posits a relationship between choice of ECT and the nurses' clinical area. Members argued that the nurses' level of knowledge is likely to affect whether or not they would select ECT as the treatment of choice. How easy would it be for nurses to recommend a treatment or intervention of which they had no or limited knowledge? Lastly, members felt that the findings section contained unsubstantiated opinions which would therefore be better located in the discussion section.

Discussion, conclusions and recommendations

In his discussion, the author argued in favour of more biological sciences to be taught in nurse education, because the 1982 syllabus and P2000 syllabus have a greater psychosocial orientation. However, earlier in his paper (p. 86) he argued that the knowledge of ECT as measured does not vary according to the qualification of the respondent. Furthermore, as stated earlier, his sample did not contain any nurses who had undergone the P2K training. It is therefore inappropriate and unwise to base arguments on such small differences when the sample does not enable potentially important comparisons to be carried out. Members expressed the view that the author appears to have an unwritten, implicit agenda, perhaps that of a return to the 'good old days' of biologically orientated nurse training, and this appears to have influenced his interpretation of the results.

Additional points included a concern regarding Pippard (1992) as a legitimate reference to support the argument regarding lack of teaching on ECT, as this was only Pippard's impression and personal opinion. Also, 'length of experience' alone may not be sufficient explanation of any existing differences. Just because some nurses may have a commonality in their length of experience since qualification does not make them a homogenous group with regard to the nature and composition of their experience. It perhaps depends on what one does with one's time during this experience.

Final comments: what meaning does this have for psychiatric and mental health nurses?

It is important for nurses who are involved with this particular treatment to be aware of the variety of issues involved in ECT. It is reasonable to suggest that the extent of a nurse's knowledge and his/her attitude towards ECT may well have an effect on how the nurse presents ECT to clients. If there are significant deficits in the nurse's knowledge of ECT, then, as the author of this research points out, there is a need to address this issue. However, the crucial point is in determining how and where this deficit can be remedied. Unfortunately, this paper does not provide enough valid findings to indicate how this deficit can be rectified.

It does raise some interesting questions for practice. One particular issue is how nurses can help clients to be fully informed (and thus give informed consent) if the nurse is unable to provide clients with all the information they need? Therefore this paper can be regarded as increasing awareness of this issue and consequently has merit.

Table 11.2 Key points arising from review No. 7.

1. The mean difference in knowledge scores was not particularly large, and no really significant differences between the groups of nurses responding existed. Yet the author's discussion said a great deal as a result of this small difference. Perhaps this raises the issue of when differences become significant and who decides.

2. Members expressed the view that the author appears to have an unwritten, implicit agenda, perhaps that of a return to the 'good old days' of biologically orientated nurse training, and this appears to have influenced his interpretation of the results.

3. The recommended changes in nurse education are not supported by the findings in the study and arguments to return to a nurse training with greater biological emphasis would need to be much more cogent and robust before such a change should be considered. However, it does raise some interesting questions for practice. In particular, how can nurses help clients to be fully informed (and thus give informed consent) when the nurses themselves are not fully informed?

References

Burnard, P. and Chapman, C. (2003) *Professional and Ethical Issues in Nursing*, 3rd edn. Baillière Tindall, London.

Cassell, C. (2004) *Essential Guide to Qualitative Methods in Organizational Research*, Sage, London.

Clarke, L. (1995) Psychiatric nursing and ETC. *Nursing Ethics*, **21**(4), 321–31.

Hammersley, M. (1992) *What's Wrong With Ethnography?* Routledge, London.

Hicks, C. (2004) *Research Methods for Clinical Therapists: Applied Project Design and Analysis*. Churchill Livingstone, Edinburgh.

Kitwood, T. and Benson, K. (1995) *The New Culture of Dementia Care*. Hawker Publications, London.

Lipson, J. (1994) The use of self in ethnographic research. In: *Qualitative Nursing Research: A Contemporary Dialogue* (ed. J. M. Morse), pp. 73–89. Sage, London.

McHale, J. and Gallagher, A. (2003) *Nursing and Human Rights*. Butterworth-Heinemann, London.

Masson, J. (1992) *Against Therapy*. HarperCollins, Glasgow.

Nolan, M., Grant, G. and Keady, J. (1997) *Understanding Family Care: a Multidimensional Model of Caring and Coping*. Open University Press, Buckingham.

Peat, J. (2002) *Health Science Research: A Handbook of Quantitative Methods*. Sage, London.

Pippard, J. (1992) Audit of electroconvulsive treatment in two National Health Service regions. *British Journal of Psychiatry*, **160**, 634.

Polit, D. F. and Hungler, B. P. (1997) *Essentials of Nursing Research: Methods, Appraisal and Utilisation*, 4th edn. Lippincott, Philadelphia.

Polit, D. F., Beck, C. T. and Hunger, B. P. (2001) *Essentials of Nursing Research: Methods, Appraisal and Utilization*, 3rd end. Lippincott, Philadelphia.

Pulsford, D. (1997) Therapeutic activities for people with dementia – what, why and... why not? *Journal of Advanced Nursing*, **26**, 704–9.

Ross, L. A. (1997) Elderly patients' perceptions of their spiritual needs and care: a pilot study. *Journal of Advanced Nursing*, **26**, 710–15.

Royal College of Nursing (1998) *Research Ethics: Guidelines for Nurses Involved in Research Or Any Investigative Project Involving Human Subjects*. Royal College of Nursing, London.

Stanfield, J. (1994) Ethnic model in qualitative research. In: *Handbook of Qualitative Research* (eds. N. Denzin and Y. S. Lincoln), pp. 175–88. Sage, London.

CHAPTER 12

The fourth stage of the **NPNR** Journal Club development: critiquing with a degree of confidence

Example 17: The NPNR National Journal Club: review from the 9th meeting

The paper reviewed was Morrison, E. F. (1990) The tradition of toughness: a study of non-professional nursing care in psychiatric nursing settings. *Image: Journal of Nursing Scholarship*, **22**, 32–8.

Abstract/overview

This paper reports on an exploratory study that attempted to identify aspects of the care organisation that may affect the violent behaviour of clients. Having noted that violence in psychiatric settings is a significant problem, the author pointed out that there was a dearth of literature that examined the influence of the organisation in relation to violent client behaviour. Using grounded theory method, a theory of non-professional nursing care was induced which had the core variable entitled 'the tradition of toughness'. Further social norms and roles were identified that operationalised the theory. The norms were (a) the need for physical restraint and (b) 'It's not you we don't trust'. The nursing roles 'enforcing' included the strategies 'policing', 'supermanning' and 'putting on a show'.

Title

Feedback comments from the members were mostly favourable. The title was regarded to be explicit and concise. Perhaps the inclusion of the word *violence* would have added to the clarity and it might have been worthwhile for the title to say what type of study it was. For example, the title could have stated that it was a grounded theory study. However, the title was felt to capture the imagination of the reader.

Abstract

Even though it wasn't titled, the paper did contain a succinct abstract (perhaps the absence of a title to the abstract was an idiosyncrasy of the particular journal and not an oversight on the part of the author). Members felt that the abstract contained the essential components of the paper and therefore gave the reader the necessary synopsis. Criticisms included the view that the abstract may have been a little brief and said very little about the methodology. Additionally, a summary of the main discussion points arising could have strengthened the abstract.

Introduction

Feedback about the introduction was predominantly favourable. The introduction was felt to set the relevant background to the study and identified the then current 'gaps' in the theory. The introduction contained a definition of violence (which appeared to be the definition of violence provided by the American Psychiatric Association in 1974), and the members' response to this definition was mixed. Some members expressed that since violence is such a subjective phenomenon, i.e. what one individual regards as violent, another would regard as assertive (Cutcliffe, 1999), the definition provided can be regarded as imprecise. However, other members felt that having a definition was necessary for the study, in that in order to explore the social processes involved in violence within certain psychiatric health care settings, it may be necessary to have an understanding of what is meant by the term 'violence'.

An alternative view was posited that suggested it was not necessary for a precise definition, in that the researcher can work with whatever conceptualisations of violence the interviewees used. Indeed, in one of his many texts on grounded theory methodology, Glaser (1992) declared that the grounded theorist approaches the area of study with only an abstract wonderment of what is going on. Yet it is also worth noting that in this day and age, where economics and the drive towards evidence-based practice have a significant influence on the research agenda within health care, justifiable concerns and/or questions could be raised of a researcher who attempted to begin a study by stating that they have an interest in a particular area but no concept of what they should be researching. Indeed, the process of writing a research proposal currently inhibits potential researchers from making such a decision. Consequently, it is perhaps no surprise that the members' feedback to the inclusion of such a definition in a grounded theory study was diverse.

Members did express some concerns that the introduction appeared to be blended with the literature review section. Given that the author used a grounded theory methodology, and Glaser and Strauss's (1967) position on the use of literature prior to commencing data collection, it would have been appropriate for the author to justify the use of a review of the literature at this stage in the study. Furthermore, as a result of this literature review it might have been prudent for the author to state that a modified version of grounded theory was used, and not grounded theory (Glaser, 1992; Cutcliffe, 2005).

Methods

Members stated that as the author was investigating an area of practice where little theory existed, the use of a grounded theory method was appropriate. The choice of obtaining data from three different settings raises the issue of the choice between a wide diverse sample or a more 'focused', narrow, concentrated sample in grounded theory. Arguments in favour of the use of a wide, diverse sample suggest that this method ensures extensive data that cover the wide ranges of behaviour in varied situations (Lincoln and Guba, 1985; Munhall and Boyd, 1993).

Another point of view could be constructed that reasons in favour of a narrower or more focused sample, rather than maximum variation. Since in grounded theory the researcher is concerned with uncovering the situated, contextual, core and subsidiary social processes, the processes need to be shared and experienced by the individuals who make up the social group. Otherwise, if an individual has no experience of the social or psychosocial process, how can they comment on it? Indeed, Lincoln and Guba (1985) pointed out that grounded theory has been termed 'local theory', as it brings together and systematises isolated, individual theory. Selection of a sample of participants who have only a limited experience of the process, or put another way, a sample that is not local, will only provide data and a subsequent theory that has a partial or limited understanding of the process being studied. Consequently, in the paper reviewed it is possible that the emerging theory amalgamates the commonalities of three local theories, each one belonging to each individual ward. Additional member comments point out that it might have been interesting too if the observation of the ward staff had been carried out covertly. Additionally, further related insights might have been gained by interviewing senior figures in the organisation (e.g. nurse managers, policy makers) and medics, although it was noted that such individuals may well be regarded as falling outside of the particular social process under investigation.

The section titled 'Setting', contained a thorough description of the people and places of the hospitals. Members indicated that this section contained some judgements on the part of the author which could have been supported or substantiated by including references/evidence. However, some examples of these judgements are included.

Ethical considerations

Members stated that the paper reported that formal access had been granted by the academic institution's human subjects committee and the hospital institutional review board. As the members were not familiar with the nuances of gaining ethical approval for a research study in an American hospital, they were unable to ascertain whether or not the correct and proper ethical considerations have been deliberated upon. Furthermore, the author indicates that individual consent was gained from each participating client.

Subjects

More detail on how the sample was selected may have been useful. In particular, members wondered if the author had used theoretical sampling, as this would have been in keeping with the methodology (Glaser and Strauss, 1967; Glaser, 1992). It is possible that the author felt that, having made it clear that she was using grounded theory, readers would automatically assume that this included theoretical sampling. Nevertheless, some additional information regarding the sampling choices indicated by the emerging theory may have been useful. The paper contains some information regarding the evolution/development of the interview content, which is also appropriate for grounded theory.

Analysis

Members reported how the author makes it clear how the different sources of data provided information on different issues. This triangulation of data sources can be perceived to add to the confirmation and completeness of the research findings (Nolan and Behi, 1995; Begley, 1996; Farmer, 2006), an argument supported by Redfern and Norman (1994), who posit that a specific advantage of using a triangulated study in nursing relates to the increased confidence in the results and a more complete understanding of the domain or process. The means to establish the credibility of the findings were rigorous and that is to the betterment of the paper. One of the methods used was to verify the truthfulness of a patient's account of an incident. In the cases where the stories were corroborated, one could argue that the truthfulness is enhanced. Where the stories were not corroborated, data was not used. A possible outcome of using this method of corroboration is that even though the client's story was true and may have added to the in-depth understanding, where the story was not corroborated, the data was not used.

The author states that she enlisted the help of two 'external experts or consultants' in order to carry out external audits and an ongoing critique of the theoretical process. According to Cutcliffe and McKenna (1999) and Angen (2000) this approach as a method of establishing the credibility of qualitative research findings has several philosophical and epistemological difficulties. Firstly, since qualitative studies are normally indicated when there is an absence of theory pertaining to the specific phenomenon or area of study being examined, how likely is it that such 'experts or consultants' will exist? Indeed, the author justifies the need for this study, in part, due to the dearth of studies in the specific area. Furthermore, the author fails to describe what defined these individuals as experts or whether they have been subjected to any criteria in order to determine the extent of their alleged expertise. If such individuals do exist, this leads to the second difficulty (Cutcliffe and McKenna, 1999). The processes of data analysis and theory induction in grounded theory depend upon the creative processes between the researcher and the data (Glaser, 1978; Glaser, 1992; Munhall and Boyd, 1993). It is unlikely then that two or more people will interpret the data in the same way or induce precisely the same categories/core variable.

Findings

Feedback from the members indicated that the findings were presented in a clear and well-structured style which included illuminating and interesting insights into the social processes which were present on the unit. These findings contained rich description and analysis supported by statements from the interviewees. The findings highlighted how the culture of the units and the nurses populating the units had a clear influence on the resulting (violent) behaviour of the clients. The abuse of the power inherent in the institution by certain individuals perpetuates the incidence of violence. Since this study was carried out in the USA and used a qualitative method, it would be inappropriate to generalise these findings. It is possible that the behaviours and social processes witnessed on the psychiatric unit are indicative of a wider cultural phenomenon; perhaps a national cultural phenomenon that encourages the 'tradition of toughness'. (This might be evidenced by such cultural norms as the constitutional right to bear arms, or the 'Hollywood'-perpetuated image of masculinity.)

However, Glaser and Strauss (1967) asserted that substantive theories are usually induced from the data and formulated first, and then these substantive theories are followed by formal theories. Consequently, as the conceptual generality of the grounded theory moves from substantive to formal theory, the scope of the theory is widened. Therefore there may well be elements of the theory induced from an American psychiatric unit that resonate with nurses from other countries and other psychiatric units.

Indeed, the findings in this paper are echoed in the experiences of many psychiatric/mental health nurses from around the world, where some nurses are allowed to behave in an inappropriate manner. Some of the members reported having witnessed similar processes within Australian psychiatric units, British psychiatric units and British Secure Hospitals (Smith and Hart, 1994; Crichton, 1995; Harbourne, 1996; Rees and Lehane, 1996; Whittington and Wykes, 1996).

Discussion, conclusions and recommendations

Members noted that the discussion highlighted the relevant supporting empirical literature and discussed the implications of the findings. It should be noted that the conclusions and recommendations were presented under the discussion heading and members felt that there may have been merit in presenting each of these in separate sections.

Final comments: what meaning does this have for psychiatric and mental health nurses?

Feedback from the group members suggested they felt this was a clear, comprehensive, interesting and illuminating paper, which highlighted an important aspect of clinical practice. Furthermore, it added to the empirical evidence in this area (and stimulated a great deal of debate in the journal clubs).

Even though the paper is of a recognised vintage, it draws attention to fundamental behaviours and dynamics within mental health care systems that need consideration and addressing. The findings (and similar experiences echoed by some of the members) suggest that the practice of some P/MH nurses appears to remain embedded and strongly influenced by the medical model. The paper reiterates that many clients with mental health problems continue to be medicalised and it reminds us of the inherent capability of a 'care system' to be more concerned with exerting power and control over the people it is supposed to be caring for. It reminds P/MH nurses of the issue of empowerment. If P/MH nurses are genuinely concerned with empowering clients, then these findings serve as a crucial and valuable insight into a mode of practice that needs to be abandoned as a matter of urgency. In addition to a culture that appears to perpetuate and glorify a 'tradition of toughness', it perhaps highlights the discomfort that some P/MH nurses may have with the expression of certain emotions, e.g. anger and frustration. In addition to these clinical issues, despite the vintage of the paper, it serves as a good example of one way of writing a qualitative research study report. Additionally, the paper contains rigorous attempts to establish the credibility or authenticity of the qualitative findings, and such endeavours are to the betterment of the paper. However, it should be noted that the technique of enlisting external experts, used by the author, has several philosophical and epistemological difficulties.

Table 12.1 Key points arising from review No. 9.

1. The paper reiterates that many clients with mental health problems continue to be medicalised and it reminds us of the inherent capability of a 'care system' to be more concerned with exerting power and control over the people it is supposed to be caring for.

2. It serves as a crucial and valuable insight into a mode of practice that needs to be abandoned as a matter of urgency and at the same time, despite the vintage of the paper, serves as a good example of one way of writing a qualitative research study report.

3. The paper contains rigorous attempts to establish the credibility or authenticity of the qualitative findings, and such endeavours are to the betterment of the paper. However, the technique of enlisting external experts, used by the author, has several philosophical and epistemological difficulties.

References

Angen, M. J. (2000) Evaluating interpretive inquiry: reviewing the validity debate and opening the dialogue. *Qualitative Health Research*, **10**(3), 378–95.

Begley, C. M. (1996) Using triangulation in nursing research. *Journal of Advanced Nursing*, **24**, 122–8.

Crichton, J. (1995) The response to psychiatric inpatient violence. In: *Psychiatric Inpatient Violence: Risk and Response* (ed. J. Crichton). Duckworth, London.

Cutcliffe, J. R. (1999) Qualified nurses' lived experience of violence perpetrated by individuals suffering from enduring mental health problems: a hermeneutic study. *International Journal of Nursing Studies*, **36**, 105–16.

Cutcliffe, J. R. (2005) Adapt or adopt: developing and transgressing the methodological boundaries of grounded theory. *Journal of Advanced Nursing*, **51**(4), 421–8.

Cutcliffe, J. R. and McKenna, H. P. (1999) Establishing the credibility of qualitative research findings: the plot thickens. *Journal of Advanced Nursing*, **30**(2), 374–80.

Farmer, T. (2006) Developing and implementing a triangulation protocol for qualitative health research. *Qualitative Health Research*, **16**(3), 377–94.

Glaser, B. G. (1978) *Theoretical Sensitivity*. Sociology Press, Mill Valley, CA.

Glaser, B. G. (1992) *Basics of Grounded Theory Analysis: Emerging vs. Forcing*. Sociology Press, Mill Valley, CA.

Glaser, B. G. and Strauss, A. L. (1967) *The Discovery of Grounded Theory: Strategies for Qualitative Research*. Aldine, New York.

Harbourne, A. (1996) Challenging behaviour in older people: nurses' attitudes. *Nursing Standard*, **12**(11), 39–43.

Lincoln, Y. S. and Guba, E. G. (1985) *Naturalistic Inquiry*. Sage, London.

Munhall, P. L. and Boyd, C. O. (1993) *Nursing Research: A Qualitative Perspective*, 2nd edn. National League for Nursing Press, New York.

Nolan, M. and Behi, R. (1995) Triangulation: the best of all worlds? *British Journal of Nursing*, **14**(10), 587–90.

Redfern, S. J. and Norman, I. J. (1994) Validity through triangulation. *Nurse Researcher*, **2**(2), 41–56.

Rees, C. and Lehane, M. (1996) Witnessing violence to staff: a study of nurses' experiences. *Nursing Standard*, **11**(13–15), 45–7.

Smith, M. E. and Hart, G. (1994) Nurses' responses to patient anger: from disconnecting to connecting. *Journal of Advanced Nursing*, **20**, 643–51.

Whittington, R. and Wykes, T. (1996) An evaluation of staff training in psychological techniques for the management of patient aggression. *Journal of Clinical Nursing*, **5**, 257–61.

Example 16: The NPNR National Journal Club: review from the 10th meeting

NB: The following review comments were originally compiled by Ian Beech, Ann Fothergill and Ben Hannigan, University of Wales.

The paper reviewed was Cutcliffe, J. R. (1999) Qualified nurses' lived experience of violence perpetrated by individuals suffering from enduring mental health problems: a hermeneutic study. *International Journal of Nursing Studies*, **36**, 105–16.

Abstract/overview

This paper reports on a study that attempted to discover the lived experiences of nurses who experience violence perpetrated by individuals suffering from enduring mental health problems. Consequently, it adopted a hermeneutic, phenomenological method which produced an emerging theory comprised of the three key themes: 'personal construct of violence', 'feeling equipped', and 'feeling supported'. As a result of his findings, the author suggested relationships between exposure to violent incidents and the ability to deal with incidents therapeutically and described how formal support systems influence this relationship.

Title

There was a mixed view from the reviewers on whether or not the title adequately explained the content and focus of the paper. The majority agreed that the title gave a clear indication of what the paper was about; however, some groups felt that it was too long and 'jargonistic'. Suggested alternatives included, replacing 'hermeneutic' with 'phenomenological' or 'qualitative'. Counter-arguments noted that if these terms were used, some criticism could be levelled at the title for not offering a precise description.

Abstract

There were some mixed views of the abstract. Many members thought that the abstract was good, in that it was concise, clearly written and gave an adequate overview of the study. Others, however, wanted more of the detail of the study, whilst some described the abstract as 'jargonistic'. Those who felt this added that it could have been strengthened by the addition of further information. For example, some members wanted more background information on the sample and explanations on the meaning of some of the concepts used in the paper. However, it is likely that giving this level of detail would have been difficult given abstract word limitations.

Introduction

Generally, members felt that the introduction to the paper was a good one. A sound justification for the study was given, and previous literature was presented and discussed. There was agreement that finding out about the experiences of nurses in relation to violence was an important topic which merited research investigation. Violence within the National Health Service remains a significant cause for concern. This concern has been reiterated recently by the United Kingdom Department of Health, which requires all National Health Service (NHS) Trusts to monitor and act to reduce violence against staff (Turnbull and Paterson, 1999) and it is reasonable to suggest that 'quick fix' solutions do not appear to be the answer. Clearly, what is needed is a deeper and more thorough understanding of the variables and interrelationships involved, in order to construct effective, workable and affordable strategies and interventions.

Methodology

The study was identified as being based on a hermeneutic phenomenological approach. The majority of members experienced difficulty understanding the philosophy used and felt that a clearer description of what phenomenology and hermeneutics are was needed. Most members were unclear about the relationship between the section of the paper which discussed phenomenological philosophy and the research study. Other groups, however, felt that the phenomenological approach added to the overall precision and clarity of the method. Several key authors (Glaser, 1978; Lincoln and Guba, 1985; Morse, 1991; Hammersley, 1992; Streubert and Carpenter, 1999) have argued that methodological precision is a hallmark of high-quality research. Thus, failure to include such precise descriptions may result (quite correctly) in criticism of the paper. However, it is incumbent upon the researcher to include clear descriptions and explanations of the method and consequently, not only address issues of methodological rigour, but additionally, increase the 'readability' and/or 'accessibility' of the paper.

Data collection

Data were collected in this study using 'semi-structured conversations'. Some members commented favourably on the attention given in the paper to the description of this method, and were particularly pleased to see the inclusion of questions used in the study. The method was felt to be congruent with the aims of the research. However, some members wanted the author to more clearly demonstrate how the use of a hermeneutic approach was reflected in his research questions, design and analysis. Whilst acknowledging that there is no one singular 'correct' way to write a qualitative research report (Dreher, 1994) members felt that the strength of the author's 'methodology and research design' section was the detailed account given of what he did and how he did it. For example, the author was praised for giving details of questions used to start each of the semi-structured conversations. Some members felt that the strengths and limitations of the method needed to be included here.

Sample

Many groups commented on the sample used in the study. The sample was chosen from a ward in which staff had experienced an unusually high level of violence. Some members felt, in this respect, that the study participants would not have been typical of most P/MH nurses. However, since nomothetic generalisation of the findings from representative populations to wider populations is not the purpose in qualitative research (Morse and Field, 1995; Morse, 1998), perhaps the selection of a sample who can provide the richest and deepest understanding of the phenomenon/process is a reasonable choice. Some members reflected this viewpoint when they commented that the paper included a good account of why this unit had been chosen.

Perhaps an alternative strategy for sampling might have been to access a P/MH population who experience a more 'usual' level of violence and gain an understanding of their 'lived experiences' of violence first. Following this, the lived experiences of P/MH nurses who experience the unusually high level of violence could be obtained, and a comparison of the two emerging theories may indicate some useful insights.

For example, further understanding of the proposed relationship between exposure to violence, the number/severity of incidents encountered, the level of support and the subsequent level of stress and/or experiential learning. All those who participated in the interviewing were described as having been full-time qualified mental health nurses. For some, the study would have been strengthened by the inclusion of unqualified nurses, and part-time staff.

Ethical considerations

There were differences of opinion with respect to the ethical dimensions of the study. Some members were critical over what they saw as a general lack of attention to this area, whilst others praised the study for the attention given to the process through which informed consent was obtained. Since ethical committee approval is required when the study occurs within NHS property (Beauchamp and Childress, 1994; Royal College of Nursing, 1998) it would have been necessary to gain ethical approval prior to conducting this study (McHale and Gallagher, 2003; Burnard and Chapman, 2003). The absence of such approval can be regarded as a deficiency of this study.

Findings

There was general praise for the systematic way in which data were analysed. Members commented on the detail given to the description of the process of thematic analysis. One group added that this level of detail was relatively rare in reports of qualitative studies. The main findings were presented around three key themes: 'personal construct of violence', 'feeling equipped' and 'feeling supported'. Some members commented favourably on the use of data extracts to illustrate the themes. A number of the groups expressed the view that the figures used to illustrate the possible relationship between clinical supervision and stress caused by experiencing violence were unhelpful, and did not clarify the points that were being made.

For some members, the findings added little in the way of new knowledge. As one group put it, 'we already knew this'. Others, however, took the view that the fact that the findings were in keeping with what was already known about the experience of violence added to their 'face validity', and that a 'lived experience' of violence had been arrived at. Some members felt that this type of study is valuable for P/MH nursing; in that they make explicit elements of theory which are implicit in the practice of many P/MH nurses. Several authors have identified the need for nursing research to shift its attention away from quantitative studies onto uncovering the unique knowledge embedded in nursing practice. According to Pearson (1992, p. 222):

> much of our scholarly theorising is only distantly related to the real world of practising nurses, especially when it utilises the most rigorous methods of positivism, the mechanistic application of problem solving or attempts to reduce or categorise the phenomena encountered in nursing.

Benner (1984) made similar remarks, asserting the need for a new paradigm of nursing research that is concerned with understanding the knowledge embedded in clinical expertise and inducing theory from this knowledge. Such theory is central to the advancement of nursing practice and the development of nursing science. Consequently, studies of this type appear to be making some attempt towards uncovering the unique knowledge embedded in P/MH nursing practice.

Many of the groups discussed the contribution of the paper to clinical practice. Whilst some felt that not much new had come from the study, others felt that this research strengthened the case for education and training. In particular, the need for greater attention to training and clinical supervision with regard to the management of violence was identified. Other members felt that the paper highlighted the need for formal policies to be implemented in the workplace in order to have comprehensive strategies for dealing with violence, debriefing and staff support.

Final comments: what meaning does this have for psychiatric and mental health nurses?

Members felt that the paper addressed an important and interesting topic which had relevance for P/MH nurses. For some, however, the paper was marred by what they saw as too much jargon and a lack of succinctness. The issue of the overuse of jargon within the NHS has been raised recently (Buggins, 1995; Casey, 1995; McGlade et al., 1996), culminating in the establishment of a nationwide group that has the remit of examining the language used by health professionals and considering the implications of this language for clients and their carers (see Buggins, 1995). More recently, Scott (1998) drew attention to the overuse of jargon within nursing, and suggested that jargon can be regarded as the language of the insecure. While the issues surrounding the use of jargon in nursing are not immediately and totally transferable to nursing research, there are parallels and consequently lessons to be learned. If a research report contains so much jargon that the potential audience it intends to reach are repelled, then the impact of the research paper on practitioners (and practice) is likely to be diminished. However, as stated previously, precise description of the research method is a hallmark of quality, and thus writers of research reports may need to include some terminology in an attempt to provide this precision. It appears that a balance of these positions should be aimed for and that the result of this may be methodologically precise research reports that reach the widest possible audience.

References

Beauchamp, T. L. and Childress, J. F. (1994) *Principles of Biomedical Ethics*, 4th edn. Oxford University Press, Oxford.

Benner, P. (1984) *From Novice to Expert: Excellence and Power in Clinical Nursing Practice*. Addison-Wesley, Menlo Park, CA.

Buggins, E. (1995) Communications: mind your language *Nursing Standard*, **10**(1), 21–2.

Burnard, P. and Chapman, P. (2003) *Professional and Ethical Issues in Nursing*, 3rd edn. Baillière Tindall, London.

Table 12.2 Key points arising from review No. 10.

1. Whilst the paper raises some interesting points and perhaps indicates several possible directions for future research, the model presented and subsequently tested (in part) in the paper was felt to be somewhat simplistic and provided little understanding of the complex interplay of processes, dynamics and variables which appear to be involved in client violence, nurses' behaviours and nurses' feelings.

2. The paper addresses an important substantive issue and considered to be 'brave' for its willingness to broach these potentially awkward and often emotive subjects such as client violence and the nurse's role in perpetuating this violence.

3. The paper contains important implications for psychiatric/mental health nursing practice, yet these were largely implicit in the paper, and perhaps would have benefited from being made explicit and from undergoing a more rigorous discussion.

Casey, A. (1995) Standard terminology for nursing: results of the *Nursing Times* Project. *Health Informatics*, **1**, 41–3.

Dreher, M. (1994) Qualitative research methods from the reviewer's perspective. In: *Critical Issues in Qualitative Research Methods* (ed. J. M. Morse), pp. 281–97. Sage, London.

Glaser, B. G. (1978) *Theoretical Sensitivity*. Sociology Press, Mill Valley, CA.

Hammersley, M. (1992) *What's Wrong with Ethnography?* Routledge, London.

Lincoln, Y. S. and Guba, E. G. (1985) *Naturalistic Enquiry*. Sage, London.

McGlade, L. M., Milot, B. A. and Scales, J. (1996) Eliminating jargon, or medicalese, from scientific writing. *American Journal of Clinical Nursing*, **64**(2), 256–7.

McHale, J. and Gallagher, A. (2003) *Nursing and Human Rights*. Butterworth-Heinemann, Edinburgh.

Morse, J. M. (1991) Qualitative nursing research: a free for all? In: *Qualitative Nursing Research: a Contemporary Dialogue* (ed. J. M. Morse), pp. 14–22. Sage, London.

Morse, J. M. (1998) What's wrong with random selection? *Qualitative Health Research*, **8**, 733–5.

Morse, J. M. and Field, P. A. (1995) *Qualitative Research Methods for Health Professionals*, 2nd edn. Sage, London.

Pearson, A. (1992) Knowing nursing: emerging paradigms in nursing. In: *Knowledge for Nursing Practice* (eds. K. Robinson and B. Vaughan). Butterworth-Heinemann, London.

Royal College of Nursing (1998) *Research Ethics: Guidance for Nurses Involved in Research or any Investigative Project Involving Human Subjects*. RCN Publishing, London.

Scott, H. (1998) Nurses must start writing so as to be understood. *British Journal of Nursing*, **7**(14), 812.

Streubert, H. J. and Carpenter, D. R. (1999) *Qualitative Research in Nursing: Advancing the Humanistic Imperative*. Lippincott, London.

Turnbull, J. and Paterson, B. (1999) *Aggression and Violence: Approaches to Effective Management*. Macmillan, London.

PART 4

Future considerations

CHAPTER 13

Using the **NPNR** approach to critiquing for a student dissertation

In Part 1 we described the context and background to critiquing nursing research, explained the purpose of such activities and detailed the evolution of the NPNR Journal Club. In Part 2 we examined a range of approaches used to critique nursing research and each chapter identified the strengths and limitations of these approaches. Each approach was also accompanied by an example (or examples) of critiques, which are based on critiques undertaken by the NPNR Journal Club. In Part 3, the book then described the NPNR Journal Club's approach to critiquing nursing research. Since this is a developmental approach, we provided two additional examples for each of the four stages identified. Having done this, Part 4 considers the future of critiquing nursing research and attempts to locate it (and consider it) within a number of related contexts. Firstly we locate it within the context of undertaking a literature review for a student dissertation. Then we locate it within the context of the discourse surrounding the complex relationship between psychiatric/mental health nursing research and multidisciplinary, collaborative research in the formal area of 'psychiatric care' in the UK. Lastly, we consider it in the context of the discourse surrounding evidence-based mental health care in Europe.

Introduction: critical thinking, critiquing and the student dissertation

For many students the culmination of their graduate and/or postgraduate education will be their dissertation. In some cases this will be a literature review; for others a piece of research incorporating such a review. Whatever the nature of this final piece of academic work, the literature review is often the most challenging aspect for students because in many ways it requires them to work and write in a way that is less familiar to them than assignment writing. As a result, this chapter will attempt to provide the reader with a guide to using the critiquing process for an academic literature review, noting the important caveat that this form of literature review is *not* the same as a systematic review of the literature (Centre for Reviews and Dissemination, 2006).

Perhaps more importantly, the skills of critiquing provide the basis for an ability that can be taken forward into clinical practice and used throughout the reader's career. Being able to engage in critical thinking and apply it to nursing problems is one way to ensure a dynamic and progressive understanding of the way things work and how nurses can bring influence to bear upon them (Alfaro-LeFavre, 2004). Reference has been made throughout this book to the advantages of being able to critique research for its application to the work area. One of the major criticisms of many academic pursuits is that they do not offer students anything tangible at the end of their study period; to a certain extent this could be argued as being so for honours research dissertations – see for example, Reading (2002) who discusses her own problems as a Nurse Teacher trying to work out how to support students struggling with their dissertation but admits that the student at the heart of the case study she quotes probably did not know how to apply all the research theory she had been exposed to throughout her studentship. On a similar note, Rolfe (1993) was also very critical of educational systems that do not focus on giving students the power to control their own knowledge.

The experiences of the authors are that often scant attention is paid to critical thinking processes within nurse education programmes. Moreover, it is not just the ability to think critically, but even fundamental structural processes, such as referencing, that can be challenging for students and academic institutions alike. This may be because of where critiquing literature is located and how it is operationalised as an academic pursuit; most often it is within the confines of a research module (or some similar course) and not woven into and across the whole curriculum. Critiquing literature, reports, research, indeed anything that requires a measure of analytical activity, necessitates personal organisation and attention to detail. It is definitely not about being able to regurgitate what is written, but to be able to access its worth, make sense of its content and contrast it to other similar/dissimilar material. In other words, it requires intellectual maturity: organisationally, structurally and cognitively. This chapter, therefore, looks at the processes of conducting a literature review and locating the critiquing the papers within the review.

Literature reviews: the three phases approach

Literature reviews are most commonly comprised of published work (though some reviews also incorporate what is referred to as 'the grey literature', e.g. reports, unpublished papers) that is clearly relevant to your research and research question. Literature reviews can also incorporate discursive pieces, theoretical papers, book chapters and electronic literature resources. The literature review can then serve as a context: one in which your proposed study can be 'located'. It shows the gaps in the extant knowledge and it should show the cumulative nature of the knowledge generated in your substantive area (assuming that the knowledge is cumulative and that is not always the case).

Interestingly, though it is seldom stated, determining when a literature review is complete is replete with judgement calls; because one cannot review every piece of research ever written, the student has to set parameters, and in so doing set arbitrary limits on what is going to be accepted within the literature review and what is not. For some, literature reviews can be conceptualised as a series of building blocks or stepping stones; the accumulation of knowledge as demonstrated through your review of the literature should lead you logically to a refined research question and resultant research design (see also Clare, 2003).

Literature reviews are not spared from the vagaries of attention to method. While the authors do not wish to conflate the type of review described above with systematic reviews of the literature, where strict adherence to method is argued by some to indicate thoroughness and thus enhance credibility (Centre for Reviews and Dissemination, 2006), it is worthy of note that all literature reviews should use a methodological approach. It is down to the student (probably in conjunction with your supervisor) to establish, rationalise and describe the organisational framework that you use for your literature review. As with approaches to critiquing research papers, the authors would not wish to purport that there is only one way to undertake a literature review. Nevertheless, for the authors of this book, one approach to enhancing the methodological soundness of literature reviews is to have three phases:

1. Broadest level of search using carefully selected search terms, synonyms, a variety of search engines and databases that tap into possibly relevant literature from a range of disciplines.
2. Abstract level search where the reviewer reads each abstract of the selected papers and excludes/removes any inappropriate papers (e.g. papers that have no real congruence with the search terms or parameters).
3. A thorough critique, using an established approach to critiquing research papers coupled with the collation of outcomes of these reviews, producing a comprehensive description of the relevant research work along with an identification of the strengths and limitations of the extant body of knowledge.

Identifying search parameters

This is the aspect of your literature review that establishes, rationalises and describes the organisational framework. In essence, this is where the student makes a number of judgement calls which set the limits of what will and will not be included and offers explanations for these choices (perhaps as a form of data trail that thus allows for replication of the review; for some this is regarded as a 'hallmark' of high quality).

The parameters that you may need to consider include:

- The age limit of the paper (i.e. what year the paper was published; e.g. papers published from 1980 until the present day will be included).
- The language the paper is written in (e.g. papers written in English and French only).
- The type of journal(s) the paper was published in.
- Empirical research papers only, or do you include theoretical and discursive papers, book chapters etc.?
- The key words you are going to use for your search.
- The search engine(s) and hard copy data sources that you are going to include.
- Whether or not you include non-peer reviewed papers.
- Whether or not you include editorials, commentaries etc.
- And whether or not the key terms are actually featured/discussed in some detail or are only mentioned briefly.

Searching for literature specifically on the subject/question you seek may only identify a small number of studies; often the information you require is spread across literature from various academic disciplines, professional groups or applications. This means that it may be hidden beneath difficult titles or associations that are, to the searcher, initially unrecognisable. For example, you are hoping to find material related to the attitudes of young people towards mental health problems. Your search is likely to need to examine literature emanating from medicine, psychology, social work, sociology, possibly social geography, and maybe anthropology. It is unlikely to be encapsulated within P/MH nursing. Broadening your search will provide you with the necessary areas of study that fit together to give you a broader picture of the primary focus. It can be thought of as similar to producing an impressionist painting; the use and blending of more than one colour helps produce a more multi-layered and stimulating product. Bringing together the disparate elements of your review into focus will enable a far more enlightened view of the whole picture, not just a narrow, introspective observation that ignores the interconnected positions of the primary positions within the knowledge base(s). The more source material there is to work with, the more chance the student has to be able to speak authoritatively about existing strengths/gaps, make comparisons and construct logical arguments.

Organising your source material

Having decided upon your parameters the next thing is to gather that material together. However, there are certain pitfalls that need to be considered during this phase of the work. It is very easy to start becoming possessive about papers as they start to accumulate on your desk. After all, having taken the trouble to find all this material, why should you even consider doing anything but keeping it all? Not only that, but having collected it you also feel the necessity to read it too – except that within the time frame available this is an impossibility; it is also unnecessary, as (our experience suggests) some papers that do fit within your literature review parameters will not have much (any) conceptual congruence with your intended research. Hence the highly pragmatic Phase 2, wherein abstracts are read to ensure that the paper does indeed speak to your substantive issue. Here are a few guiding principles.

Try to:

- Store the material under the disciplinary/substantive areas in which you have collected them. This can be either hard or virtual copy, depending on where it came from. It will serve you well to know where material is once you have obtained it. Poor storage and filing is a key to disaster. There is no right or wrong way to do this: develop a system that suits you and enables you to access your literature easily.
- Design a reading record so that each time you start to read one of your papers you have information about the key points you read at hand. It can be frustrating for you having read something you consider to be very important for you only to discover three months later that you cannot remember which paper it was in, and therefore cannot reference it in your review.
- Know when material is coming in to you. For example, you may be 'hand searching' hard copies and therefore collecting material as you go along. However, it is also likely that your librarian is collecting material you have requested and you need to know when this will arrive. It can be frustrating thinking that you have everything ready for your critique only for another set of papers to come in that need screening.
- Regularly discuss the material you are reading, critiquing, screening etc. with others, specifically your supervisor. It is much easier to test views, opinions and analysis if you rehearse it on a regular basis. Of course, it is

also very useful for your supervisors too, because it gives them an opportunity to explore your thoughts as you progress and the material from which you are developing them. It can be very difficult for a supervisor to make sense of your arguments if they are unaware of your sources. It can also reduce the amount of work and/or rewriting necessary because drafts can be prepared in the knowledge that there is already agreement about the nature of the debate.

- Track your references so that you can get to the source of other authors' conclusions. It is not uncommon for people to misquote material from their own sources, or even to draw the wrong conclusions from something they have read. If you perpetuate this in your own work, and others do the same thing, it means that something that is inacuurate is being substantiated and will, eventually, become the accepted position. Not only is this bad for you, especially if your supervisors and/or assessors know different, but also for nursing generally because it means that they are basing elements of their theoretical underpinnings on false or suspect research findings. Knowing that you are quoting from the original source should give you more confidence in your arguments. And, if what you read in that original source conflicts what others have said about it subsequently, this adds further credence to your own critique.
- Discard anything that you do not need
- Set time limits on the different parts of the process – for example a month to gather the main sections of the source material and a further month to track down original articles. Agree arrival times with your librarian.
- Lastly, even though this is not necessarily part of the organisational process, get to know the correct referencing approach expected by your academic institution. By doing so you will store the material, especially from sources other than books and journals, in a way that is both organisationally correct as well as being easy for you to trace should you need to do so. Internet addresses and personal communications are classic examples of these.

Try not to:

- Leave your source material lying around un-filed. You can guarantee that you will misplace it, and you will only realise it just when you need it.
- Commit everything to memory. No one can keep all this information in their head, especially as in many cases you are not yet making real sense of it and therefore cannot really understand what it is all about. We remember things in different ways, but can only commit information to memory so that it can be successfully recalled if it somehow makes sense to us. You will not be able to remember everything that you have read, so do not try. Trust in your developed storage system.
- Read your literature without writing your thoughts down at the same time.
- Collect duplicates.

- Get creative! When you start collecting material it is very easy to let your imagination wander. If it becomes increasingly difficult to find the literature that you are looking for it becomes attractive to collect that which is more readily available. You convince yourself that collecting papers that have a tenuous link to one of your already minor sources is really important. It isn't, and all it will do is deflect you from the real work.
- Keep literature that you have already screened as being unsuitable. It is all too easy to be attracted to reviewing papers just because they are there. Being available does not increase the robustness or suitability of a piece of literature. The review process is involved and requires careful consideration. Clouding issues with papers that do not fit and then having to edit them out of a argument or proposition is simply increasing the pressure.

The above represent the activities that are necessary in the first two phases of your literature review. Next we consider the necessity of critique as the pivotal process of Phase 3. It is important to note here that the level of detail of a student's critique may very well depend upon the level of academic program that he/she is engaged upon. Indeed, some provision for this variation in level of rigour and detail exists in the approaches (see for example Burns and Grove (1993, Chapter 4)). That being said, the authors view it as axiomatic that the more rigorous and detailed the level of critique and the greater the student's familiarity with the extant literature, the more the student will be conversant with the epistemological and methodological nuances of the studies related to the substantive issue being considered and the greater the chance of not repeating the limitations inherent in existing studies.

Critiquing the literature

To reiterate, a review of the literature should include some form of critique or critical reading of the extant work; merely describing what exists already is inappropriate. This is a common limitation of literature reviews undertaken by students and yet, even allowing for variation in academic level, this critique must be evident. To a greater or lesser extent, depending on the academic level of the student, the literature review should make reference to the theoretical, methodological, ethical substantive and presentational strengths and weaknesses of the papers. In other words, the overall critique of the body of literature is mirrored by the critique of individual papers. Thus, as the student critiques individual pieces of work, this then enables a critical perspective on the body of knowledge, and as a consequence a more robust and accurate rationale for the research question, to be obtained.

Prudence dictates that the authors of this book acknowledge that the depth and detail of critique in a student's literature review is going to be driven or influenced by the particular requirements of the academic program upon which the student is engaged. To paraphrase, the depth of critique from an under-graduate student who is undertaking a literature review as the culmination of his/her degree is likely to be more 'shallow' than a critique of the literature which occurs as a prelude to a research study for a PhD. Nevertheless, as highly experienced examiners of student literature reviews of various academic levels (from baccalaureate to PhD), the authors of this book would expect to see some evidence of the following in a literature review:

- Has the student made some reference to the theoretical, substantive, meth-odological, ethical and presentational dimensions of either the collection of papers or each individual paper?
- Has the student considered whether or not the reviewed work points to or suggests the next logical research question(s) to be asked?
- Has the student indicated whether the literature indicates that the research that has been undertaken thus far has a cumulative, sequential progressive focus or has more of a sporadic, disparate look to it? This point needs fur-ther explanation. Literature reviews should examine the body of work in the substantive area for evidence of cumulative, longitudinal knowledge genera-tion: evidence of what has been termed the 'incremental change of routine science' (see Gamota, 2006). Notwithstanding the value of what have been termed 'discontinuous change or scientific revolutions' (Gamota, 2006), evi-dence that studies have not built upon what is already known (and similarly, not bridged gaps in the extant literature) would have major implications for the accumulation of knowledge in the substantive area. This means that building solid, mid-range theory is problematic if not completely thwarted. Unfortunately, and while not wishing to be indecorous or harsh, missing the longitudinal nature of knowledge generation is perhaps indicative of a more endemic, epistemological phenomenon in nursing research *per se*. In her fine scholarly paper, Meleis (2002, p. 4) discovered that:

> Most reported studies continue to focus on one-project, one-centre, or one-country research endeavours instead of combining scholarly ener-gies and packaging them for multi-centre and multinational research goals that could lead to a more powerful collective voice.

Such epistemological mistakes can be avoided if the literature review consid-ers this phenomenon and thus asks logical 'next step' research questions.
- Has the student critiqued the papers in the literature review with an approach that is philosophically and methodologically congruent with the designs/methods used in each study? In other words, if one continues to critique qualitative papers using an approach that was designed for quantitative

papers, then the quality of the research will always be shown to be flawed. Inversely, if one continues to critique quantitative papers using an approach that was designed for qualitative papers, this will also indicate flaws in the research papers.

■ Has the student considered and discussed what meaning(s) or worth the study has for the practice and knowledge base of P/MH nursing?

■ Has the student included both strengths and limitations of papers?

Summary

Thus the individual critiques aggregate to help form a more complete whole that has the ability to inform the relationships between the papers. There are probably (at least) two ways of progressing at this point. The first entails making a list of the key points for the whole of the review, adjusting them so they are in the order in which you wish to present them, and then writing the review. The second is to write up each section of the search area critiques in turn, making the connections between each one as you progress. Either way, at the end of the draft writing period you are likely to have the skeleton of the review, but at least it will contain the key issues you wish to raise. It will, from your critiques, also have the key elements of a review, namely the strengths and weakness of the literature itself and the interconnected elements that come together to make cohesive and articulate arguments for undertaking your own dissertation research project. This first draft needs to have all the elements in it, but you will undoubtedly need to redraft to ensure that it reads well and answers all the questions germane to the focus of your study. This is a good time to bring in your supervisor, prior to extensive rewrites that may, or may not, be necessary.

References

Alfaro-LeFevre, R. (2004) *Critical Thinking and Clinical Judgement: a Practice Approach*, p. 136. Saunders, St Louis.

Burns, N. and Grove, S. K. (1993) *The Practice of Nursing Research: Conduct, Critique and Utilisation*, 2nd edn. W. B. Saunders, Philadelphia.

Centre for Reviews and Dissemination (recovered 2006) *Systematic Reviews*. http://www.york.ac.uk/inst/crd/crdreview.htm.

Clare, J. (2003) Writing a PhD thesis. In: *Writing Research: Transforming into Text* (eds. J. Clare and H. Hamilton), Chapter 2. Churchill Livingstone, Edinburgh.

Gamota, G. (recovered 2006) *Towards a Science-Based Framework for Developing Science Metrics*. http://www.wren.network.net/events/2003.

Meleis, A. (2002) Whither international research? *Journal of Nursing Scholarship*, **34**(1), 4–5.

Reading, S. (2002) Supporting students in undergraduate research: anxieties, ambiguities and agendas. In: *Developing Professional Judgement in Health Care: Learning Through the Critical Appreciation of Practice* (eds. D. Fish and C. Coles), pp. 139–56. Elsevier Science, Edinburgh.

Rolfe, G. (1993) Towards a theory of student-centred nurse education: overcoming the constraints of a professional curriculum. *Nurse Education Today*, **13**, 149–54.

CHAPTER 14

The future of psychiatric and mental health nursing research?

All too often researchers, and not just those working in nursing, are accused of being out of touch with the reality of what goes on in the real world. Whether this is correct or not is probably unimportant, but what is clear is that research often does not benefit from the same level of credibility as a person's own experience of the workplace. This is entirely understandable when you consider the cognitive mechanisms in place to help us frame our thought processes and decision-making activities. However, if we were to try to survive solely on our instincts within a professional arena it would not be long before we were overwhelmed with questions for which we simply did not have any answers. Trial and error may be all right for the developing child, but nurses are adults, dealing, in the main, with adult problems and as nurses we have to have access to adult solutions. It would be professionally arrogant to assume that our practical experience alone could place all the answers at our fingertips, and besides, mental health care has become so sophisticated over the last 30 years that, working exclusively from past or observed experience would gradually reduce, not increase, our body of collective knowledge. If P/MH nursing is to meet the challenge of providing appropriate and complex care it has to have more at its disposal than myth and legend. The reality is that our future success lies in combining all the evidence resources at our disposal, including research, with the spontaneity of our intuitive actions and subjecting both to the same level of critical evaluation; in short, raising the level of our professional thinking to a more mature status.

To enable this to happen certain key issues have to be addressed, and this involves more than the simplistic solution of encouraging individual practitioners to read more research, or researchers to do more practice-based projects. No, the route to success involves understanding what part the science and art of nursing have to play in this development process and attributing to them suitable responsibilities and expectations (Bekker *et al.*, 1999). In the space available to us within this chapter we cannot possibly deal with the whole of this agenda and will therefore address the part that should be played by research and evidence. We also recognise that research alone cannot function in a vacuum and that for it to be effective, reciprocal influences must come from the areas in which it is to be considered and used. Therefore we have divided the chapter into two sections: the responsibilities of research in relation to nursing and the responsibilities of nursing in relation to research.

The responsibilities of research in relation to nursing

On the face of it, any research endeavour has one major objective: to provide information that answers questions. Research linked to a professional discipline is no different. The major difference between professional researchers and those undertaking research within a profession is that in most cases researching itself will be a secondary function to some other professional role. This is not just the case within nursing. If one looks at the evidence base generated within psychiatry, it is almost exclusively the work of practising psychiatrists, and the same applies within the fields of social work and other disciplines allied to medicine. There are implications for this form of practice and we will address them later in this chapter; however, the point here is that in most cases, those undertaking discipline-related research should have a good understanding of the work of that discipline and be well grounded in the questions for which it needs answers. The main question need not necessarily be whether the researcher has the ability to link research with practice, but whether or not the research they choose to undertake is of a good enough quality to have relevancy for other practitioners. If it can be established that the design, method and robustness of the research activity reach the necessary standard, there is then the question of how, and in what form, the research reaches others for use as an intelligence source. Finally, there is the question of how that work finds its way into practice and its impact is evaluated. From these questions we can identify five themes that collectively sum up the responsibilities of research in relation to any chosen subject that it purports to represent:

1. The appropriateness of the research topic and its relevance to other members of the profession or users of their services
2. The quality of the research activity – including the identification of appropriate methods and designs
3. The coherence of the writing and dissemination strategy associated with a specific piece of research
4. The attention given to the practical application of the research and how this is expressed within the researcher's reports.
5. The effectiveness of the evaluative feedback loop between researcher and practitioner/user

These five themes will now be considered in more detail.

1. The appropriateness of the research topic

If you were asked to explain why it was that you had arrived late for work, you would be regarded with a certain amount of suspicion if you began your excuse by venturing the belief that there was life on the planet Mars. Similarly, if you were asked by an anxious relative to explain why it was that a patient who almost perpetually self harmed by using razor blades to cut tracks into her arms was being allowed the freedom to repeat such activities even though she came under the seemingly protective umbrella of in-patient care, your response would be of little use if it did not specifically address not just the question, but the concern behind its asking.

We have already stated that all too often practitioners see research as answering the wrong questions, but there is also the other issue of whether it provides the right answers. If you undertake a review of P/MH nursing research papers printed over the last 35 years, you will discover that they follow a particular trend. The intensity of that trend is more marked as we reach the current day. In the early 1970s most nurses undertaking and reporting research (though certainly by no means all) were either working as research assistants for medical staff or researching topics which were of a medical or psychiatric nature. Diagnostic activities, illness presentations and drug actions research were the domain of both medical as well as nursing staff. In the main the research methods used by both disciplines were often similar, though there was at times stark contrast between the totally quantitative approaches of psychiatry and the predominantly qualitative ones adopted by nurses. The main difference between the research activities of the two disciplines was that psychiatry was building a knowledge base that was to constitute the foundations for its present work and research activities, whilst nursing was replicating psychiatry and doing little to establish an evidence foundation upon which to build knowledge for nursing. As one comes closer to the present day we find that nursing has increasingly concentrated its efforts on researching issues that are central to the work of its own discipline. However, the legacy of those earlier years can still be seen, and the future challenge will be to re-focus nurse researchers' endeavours on nursing-related research issues (Ward *et al.*, 1999b).

The *nurse-oriented research focus* should be what drives the unidisciplinary research agenda, but it is important that nurses do not simply select nursing topics on which to concentrate (Crowe, 1998; McCabe, 2000). True, if nurses are to be recognised as equal partners within the multidisciplinary team they have to be able to articulate their own evidence in support of their decision-making activities, but to be genuine team members they need to take part in team activities. So much of contemporary psychiatry is based around group decision-making, and this has to be driven by group research. Service delivery cannot exist without nurses, and it therefore follows that nurses must be involved in the research that establishes the nature, organisation, resourcing and evaluation of that care. Equally, the care itself cannot function isolated from the work of other disciplines, so nursing research has to both dovetail and collaborate with the research activities of those disciplines. Compared with 30 years ago, perhaps the major change is that nurses must take the lead in their own research rather than allowing others to do it for them. In the case of multidisciplinary research, there is also no reason why nurses should not take the lead as long as they are suitably qualified to do so – for examples of this approach see Onyett *et al.* (1995), Ward *et al.* (1999a) and Wooff *et al.* (1988).

It would be inappropriate for us to state here what we consider to be the *research priorities* for P/MH nursing. Such things are determined by individuals, groups and organisations in relation to the local context (Barker *et al.*, 1999). There does, of course, have to be a balance between what the individual wants to do and what needs to be done; what the individual thinks is important and that which contributes to the general good; and that which develops the individual and that which develops their professional group. Such decisions should be made in collaboration with others and we would strongly recommend that no research project be undertaken solely on the strength of one individual working alone. However, within psychiatric and mental health nursing there are areas of general concern that appear to influence service thinking no matter where the individual works, and nursing research has to continue to address these issues in the future if it is to contribute to the process of defining nursing responsibilities. These include:

- Nurses' use of traditional management techniques, such as control and restraint, seclusion and PRN medications (Bowers *et al.*, 2000b; Chien, 1999; Mason, 1997; see also McDonald and Gallon, 2006; Noak *et al.*, 2006)
- The use of special observations for those who are deemed to be at risk of harming themselves or others (Cleary *et al.*, 1999; Barker and Cutcliffe, 1999; Jones *et al.*, 2000a,b; Neilson and Brennan, 2001; see also Cutcliffe and Barker, 2006; Ward and Jones, 2006))
- Risk assessment and management (Gournay and Bowers, 2000; Hazelton, 1999; Raven and Rix, 1999)
- The evaluation of psychotherapeutic interventions (Marks, 1977; Gournay *et al.*, 2000b; Reilly, 2001)
- Nurse prescribing (Allen, 1998; Gray and Gournay, 2000; Kaas *et al.*, 2000)
- The roles and responsibilities of those working as independent practitioners specifically within community settings (Atkinson, 1996; Bennett *et al.*, 1995; Wilkinson, 1992; Ward *et al.*, 1999c; Ward and Jones, 1997; White and Brooker, 2001)
- Working in different care settings, and increasingly the problems facing in-patient care (Gournay *et al.*, 1997a; Ward *et al.*, 2000)

- Working with different diagnostic and age groups (Gournay and Beadsmoore, 1995; Akhtar and Samuel, 1996; Cole *et al.*, 1996; Conrad, 1998; Barker, 1999; Stordeur *et al.*, 2000)
- Working with different ethnic and cultural groups (Rodriguez *et al.*, 1992; Lutzen and Nordin, 1995; Takeuchi and Cheung, 1998)
- Philosophical issues in relation to care (Lutzen and Nordin, 1994; Nolan *et al.*, 1998; Carlsson *et al.*, 2000; Cutcliffe and Goward, 2000)
- Clinical decision making (Carpenter, 1991; Alty, 1997; Narayan and Corcoran, 1997)
- User involvement (Valimaki *et al.*, 1996; Forchuk *et al.*, 1998; Rogers *et al.*, 1997)
- Nursing leadership (McGleish, 1996; Murrells & Robinson, 1997)
- Clinical supervision (Cutcliffe and Proctor 1998a,b, Cutcliffe *et al.*, 1998a,b; Cutcliffe and Hyrkas, 2006; Ashmore and Carver, 2000; Coffey and Coleman, 2001; Edwards *et al.*, 2000)
- Educational issues, particularly the preparation of psychiatric and mental health nurses (Hardcastle, 1999; Sainsbury Centre for Mental Health, 1997; Lakeman, 1999)
- National and international collaboration (Chiu, 1999; International Society of Psychiatric-Mental Health Nurses, 1999; White, 1998)
- The future of psychiatric and mental health nursing, including the debate concerning generic and specialist workers (Allen, 1998; Butterworth, 1991; Barker *et al.*, 1999, Cutcliffe and McKenna 2000a,b; Ward *et al.*, 1999c; see also Cutcliffe and McKenna, 2006; Younge and Boschma, 2006)

It is also important for nurse researchers to ensure that their work is appropriate to the needs of both the other nurses and service users. This should always entail discussion and decision making with others and specifically those from within the practice domain. Similarly, it is the responsibility of researchers to ensure that they are not carrying out work that has already been completed by others. There are, of course, occasions when this is important, either to establish whether the original findings were accurate or if they can be replicated in other areas or time frames. There is also the need to maintain interest in research once it has been completed. The completion of a project and the resultant scientific paper should not constitute the end of the research. Invariably research recommendations suggest that further work is needed to make more sense of the total picture, yet rarely do nurse researchers follow this through themselves. There is a need for research to be part of a programme of work, or at least to fit into an overall strategy of inquiry. Longitudinal studies are rare in nursing generally and even more so in mental health. Follow-up studies have been undertaken (Gournay *et al.*, 2000; Newell and Gournay, 1994), but again these are not often tackled. For P/MH nursing to develop its research and evidence base the research itself has to be more than just individuals 'shooting in the dark'. Establishing research priorities that give a sense of purpose to all this effort has to come from nurses and be driven by the skills of researchers. More importantly, it has to become part of the strategic thinking of nursing and its leaders, embedded in the desire to improve and accountable to a collective vision of the future. Only by coordinating our research efforts will nursing ever be able to 'join up' all our resources into an accessible body of knowledge (Butterworth, 1991).

Mental health nurses must also contribute to *multidisciplinary research* activities, otherwise the whole nature of nursing will be become insular and detached from mainstream psychiatry and care service thinking (Gournay *et al.*, 2001; Ricard, 1999). There are benefits to being a strong and relatively large minority group, but specialisation has its price. If nurses only pursue nursing research they may eventually run out of ideas, creativity and imagination (Walters, 1990). Exposure to others only enhances diversity, and so it should be if nursing research is to flourish. Areas where nurses can contribute to this agenda are only limited by the degree of commitment nurses have to it. Whether nurses take the lead on these ventures will be determined by several factors, not least the relationship between individuals and their research experience. The reality is that at present very little published material exists around the developing face of 21st century psychiatry and its organisation. The following represents a small percentage of the areas where nurses need to consider being involved, not just as practitioners but also in researching both the effectiveness and development of change.

- The development of evidence based care
- Clinical governance and quality control mechanisms generally
- Care pathways
- Service configuration
- Formal and rigorous practice development
- Mental health and human rights legislation and their implication for practice and service delivery
- Therapeutic interventions
- Multi-agency working
- Evaluations of existing service provision and establishing benchmarks for future change
- Introduction of government policy initiatives
- Clinical leadership

2. The quality of nursing research

Quality is more than establishing the right fit at the right price. In relation to research it covers a much broader set of items. It is not acceptable to say that research produced results that are viable or up to standard if we are only seeking to support our own arguments or contentions. Research has to play a far more independent role. For it to be genuinely credible it has to be impartial, not simply proving a point. Good research is designed to find out, not prove (Cutcliffe *et al.*, 2000). This can only be achieved by ensuring that the *research methods* to be used are suitable to the subject being researched: that the choice between qualitative or quantitative (or a combination of both) approaches is appropriate to the question; that the tools selected (if any) are both reliable and valid; that the sample is sufficient to produce the data necessary and that its analysis follows accepted scientific principles; that conclusions from the analysis are not driven by personal agendas; and that the shortcomings as well as the successes of the research are recorded for others to make their own judgement about its quality.

Another trend that has appeared in the P/MH nursing research literature over the last 35 years is that of the use of qualitative research. Unlike the topics themselves, which have tended to move away from psychiatry, the more contemporary literature shows a marked increase in the use of different methodologies with a definite move towards undertaking far more qualitative work, in line with psychiatry itself. Many nurse researchers now argue that nursing has become far more adult in its use of research methods and it now has enough knowledge of these to be able to use those appropriate to the study, rather than choosing studies appropriate to their knowledge (Burnard and Hannigan, 2000; Croom *et al.*, 2000; Cutcliffe and Goward, 2000). The literature itself is testimony to this, with research from P/MH nurses using any number of different approaches (Bowers *et al.*, 2000a; Carlsson *et al.*, 2000; Gournay and Bowers, 2000; Gournay *et al.*, 1997b; Tang *et al.*, 2001).

Quality can only be achieved by researchers learning from and reporting their mistakes. One way of achieving this is through *research supervision*. All too often, inexperienced researchers undertake potentially significant pieces of work without approaching other, more experienced, researchers for guidance and support. So much effort can be wasted simply for the sake of spending a little more time in preparing the study properly. Nurses who have as their main job some form of professional activity other than research carry out most of the research undertaken within psychiatric and mental health nursing. This is not the case with many other disciplines. For many of those carrying out projects the work may well be part of their own professional development, as is the case with those completing higher degrees. Certainly, these individuals are very much on the increase (Ward *et al.*, 2000), which bodes well for the future. However, the fact remains that their skills base cannot be considered to be as broad or as in-depth as those who undertake research for a living and have consequently received appropriate supervision, ongoing training and feedback about their performance. In effect, amateurs, no matter how talented, undertake most nursing research, as is the case for psychiatry, sometimes with dire consequences (Prior *et al.*, 2001). Without the proper guidance from an experienced supervisor, 'amateurish' will be the tag attributed to their work. Nursing cannot afford to be so entrepreneurial!

Sometimes, of course, the results of poorly developed research are reported in professional journals as fact, leading practitioners to consider inaccurate findings as possible drivers for their own practice. Rarely do such papers ever get past the rigorous review processes of research and scientific journals, but it is fair to say that these are not the popular day-to-day reading material of working nurses, so the likelihood of such bad science influencing change is increased. As we have already discussed at length in this book, the necessity for nurses to be able to critique both poor as well as good research is crucial if this situation is to be avoided.

3. Reporting and disseminating research

Many people find that having completed a piece of research, especially those for academic courses, they are then reluctant to write up the work for publication. There are several reasons for this: the fact that there is no longer any pressure to complete the task and it is easy to keep on saying, 'I will do it next week'; the individual may not have experience of writing for publication and the activity is a daunting one that they are not prepared to tackle; the absence of a supervisor to help with the production of a manuscript; or simply that the individual feels their work would not be of value to others. Waddell reports that too little research finds its way into print, and even then it is not read or used properly (Waddell, 2001), whilst Kempster contends that evidence-based journals are either not prepared to publish work in mental health or do not receive papers which are of a good enough standard to be published (Kempster, 1998).

It should go without saying that all research has to be published or at least made available for public consumption. If researchers keep information to themselves, even if they are unsure as to its value, it means that others cannot benefit from it. There are several questions that have to be asked when considering writing for publication and future researchers must ensure that they answer them and then follow them through.

■ Has the research project specifically allocated time at the end of the work for writing up?
■ Has the research material been prepared with a view to being easy to convert into a published paper, i.e. is it accessible?
■ How many different papers can the research support?
■ Should the paper be sent to a professional or a scientific journal, or both using different styles?

- Have the specific styles of the targeted journal been considered so that the paper can be written to their contributors' criteria?
- Has the researcher contacted the editor of the targeted journal beforehand to establish that the intended paper is appropriate and that the journal would be interested in receiving it?
- What format does the journal want the manuscript to be sent in (hard copy, email etc.), and how many copies need to be sent?
- Does the researcher need to get help from a supervisor to help write the paper?
- Have time frames been set to complete the work?
- Is there someone who can read and critique the paper before it is sent to a journal for consideration?
- Is the researcher aware that some journals are stricter than others in terms of peer review and that in many cases papers will be returned for editing, correction and, in some cases, major rewriting? If so, has time been allocated to this work?
- What happens if the paper is rejected completely?

Of course, writing for publication is only part of the dissemination process. Once work is complete it has to be championed by the researcher, those involved in the work and those who supported it. This means conference presentations and teaching sessions, and researchers have to be prepared to defend their work within those environments and, if needs be, obtain the skills to be able to do so. This is not an easy task for many people and must be taken into consideration when research is being planned. Too few inexperienced researchers appreciate that the *dissemination strategy* must be integral to any research proposal or outline and carry as much importance as the quality of the research itself.

4. The practical application of research

Whilst it may be assumed that once research has been completed, the papers written and the dissemination strategy undertaken the job of the researcher is complete, but this is not necessarily the case. Even when potential research is being considered, thought has to be given to its applicability to the practical environment and though not all research is designed for implementation, especially that of a philosophical nature, work stimulated by observations from practice certainly should be. The *implementation strategy* is often no more than the purpose of carrying out the project in the first place, though in more sophisticated programmes it will be the driving force for completing the work. In many cases the application of research into practice has to be the responsibility of the researcher, but obviously it has to involve others because culture change or practice developments cannot be successful if they do not engage all those who will be affected by it (Cutcliffe *et al.*, 1998; Jackson *et al.*, 1999a,b).

Research should not be undertaken for its own sake; we cannot afford the time to be that self-indulgent. It has to serve a purpose and in a professional environment dominated by clinical practice this must provide the rationale for such activities. Certainly practitioners need to take much of the responsibility for ensuring the quality of any research adoption, but the researcher should take an active part in the process by ensuring initially that the work undertaken provides the sort of material that those practitioners need. *Practice development* should be as rigorous as the work that underpins it, but if research outcomes are inconsistent with the demands of practice developers it is a failure of research planning (Ward *et al.*, 1998). Discussion and outcome clarification need to be undertaken at the very start of an intended project, revisited throughout its life and evaluated as part of its terminal activities.

5. Research feedback

If a piece of research is completed, published and disseminated properly the opportunities are there for the researcher to gain invaluable feedback from others about the nature of the work. These lessons have to be learnt, for as we have already described, the vast majority of P/MH nursing research is not undertaken by professional researchers. Researchers are sometimes accused of being arrogant, and much of this stems from either their unwillingness or inability to listen to what others say about the quality or appropriateness of their work. The work of the NPNR Journal Club involves just that process, and when publishing the aggregated critiques of over 500 nurses about specific published papers it would be unwise of their authors not to take note, and learn from, those reviews. In theory, nurse research should improve as we progress through this century. We have a growing body of knowledge, we have an increasing number of individuals equipped to carry out good quality and suitable research, and we have a culture that values research and evidence far more than ever before. No one expects every piece of research to be perfect – indeed very little of it ever is. What is expected is that mistakes form the basis of development and that researchers acknowledge those mistakes when presenting their findings. There is always room for improvement and professional egos should not stand in the way of progress. It has to be the responsibility of a researcher, once a project is complete, to actively seek the informed feedback of others about the nature of their work. By doing so we can expect better quality work, more individuals equipped to provide research supervision, a more focused research agenda and a better informed nursing workforce. The feedback loop, therefore, is an essential component of an upwardly spiralling quality improvement programme.

The responsibilities of nursing in relation to research

Though it is true that researchers have to take responsibility for their own research, the terminal feedback loop discussed above is not the only point at which nurses have a responsibility to support research and researchers. There are various times within both the planning and the life of projects where the involvement of those outside of the direct research process can make a genuine contribution to its success and quality. The whole purpose of this book is to bring to nursing's attention a mechanism for one form of feedback, but it is by no means the only one. Research critiquing certainly encapsulates the essence of professional awareness, but invariably it is a process carried out after the work has been completed. Indeed, it could even be argued that research papers do not tell everything about the research itself, and as such much of what goes on within the research world could still be hidden from the critical eye of nurses. It is crucial that all nurses are involved in some way or another with the development of the P/MH nursing knowledge base, because in truth it has to belong to them if it is to have any meaning. If individual nurses do not take advantage of those possibilities nurse researchers could quite rightly take the opposing view from that described at the beginning of this chapter and accuse nursing itself of being out of touch with what goes on in the real world. We have to be quite clear about this: however or wherever the evidence is gathered, developed and disseminated, the future of psychiatric and mental health nursing, along with all other disciplines delivering mental health care, will centre upon proof that its actions are the best and most appropriate for service user needs. If nurses feel removed from the source of that evidence it will be very difficult for them to take an active part in its adoption and as such will offer care which is either unsubstantiated or not of the best quality. If, by contributing to the research or evidence-generating process, nurses can get a sense that they own that knowledge for themselves then it will cease to be vested with the mystical qualities historically attributed to research activities. In doing so, evidence generation and implementation becomes a dynamic process and 21st century P/MH nursing practice the main beneficiary. Let us consider those areas where nurses can make a difference within this agenda.

1. The appropriateness of the research topic

In an ideal world each practitioner would undertake their own research work, thus rendering the necessity to communicate his or her needs to others completely superfluous. Of course, such a situation is totally impractical and would in itself be very counterproductive. However, if we examine this highly improbable situation in more detail it provides us with ideas as to what needs to be considered for non-researchers to be able maintain research quality.

Some people have to research, while others have to inform research decisions and in a reciprocal process use the research findings to inform their practice. Not everyone wants to be a researcher. Not everyone has the skills to undertake research. Not everyone has the work opportunities or allocated time to be able to commit themselves to researching. Notwithstanding this, this does not mean that research is the domain of researchers or a minority of the 50,000 plus psychiatric and mental health nurses registered in the UK alone. Being committed to research does not mean you have to undertake it, but it does mean you have to support it. It also means demystifying its language, activities and methods so that those who do not use these things regularly can at least understand what their researching colleagues are doing. The first task in maintaining quality is the ability to recognise it when you see it and that can only be achieved if you have a reasonable *knowledge of the specialist vocabulary*. As you will have seen from the review chapters, and in particular whilst exploring the different critiquing approaches, this does not mean having an intimate working knowledge of research. It means that you can picture what it is that the researcher is talking about and shape an impression of their work and intentions. It also gives some clues as to how they intend to achieve their outcomes and makes reading and understanding their findings more of a possibility. To do this it is necessary to organise your thoughts into patterns so that you concentrate on the specific aspects of the paper, looking for things that should be there and those that should not. Having some form of checklist as an *aide mémoire* is an ideal way of achieving this.

Secondly, having demystified the language you have to desensitise yourself to the fact that research is something which can only be understood by other researchers. There is a commonly held belief that research is only published for the benefit of other researchers, and this is, or at least should be, totally untrue. Research, when published, enters the public domain and is free to all who read it. Contained within those papers is the 'stuff of kings', if only their secrets could be unlocked. But this is not as difficult as it seems, as we have already shown in the previous chapters. What is important is for non-researchers to lose their suspicion of research as a 'not for them' entity. Half the battle is overcoming the psychological barrier of so-called academic snobbery. Once that has been achieved, then research, no matter in how much depth it is read, becomes far more accessible.

Thirdly, the process of communicating information is all-important. We have already considered the role of researchers writing about their research, but what we are suggesting here is something that happens long before decisions about potential projects take place. Non-researchers – in effect, practitioners – are also guilty of not writing about their clinical practice. There are any number of professional journals representing P/MH nursing to which papers about practice could be sent. Yet a brief analysis of these shows that much of what they contain centres around policy, legislation, personal views and research. Very few articles describe service structures or discuss clinical issues. This is a turnaround from the situation 35 years ago when the vast majority of these articles addressed just such issues. Nurses need to *write about their clinical practice* for researchers to have an anchor or benchmark to begin the inquiry. For many researchers this is where their ideas about research activities come from.

For others the ideas come from discussions, collaboration, practice links and supervision. But these too are the responsibility of other nurses. If, as we have suggested, most researchers in nursing have some link with the clinical base, then it is the conversations that occur within them that shape people's thoughts and ideas about the subject matter for their intended research. Equally, when research has been published, all too often, having read a paper, nurses will think to themselves that this was inappropriate or could have been done in a different way that would have been more beneficial to them. *Writing to the journal* is one way of registering this fact, and all journals have a letters section. The fact is that nurses need to be more proactive in their support of research and lodge their dissatisfaction at what they see as being invalid. If no one tells a journal that what they published is not what they want, then the journal has no way of knowing this except through its circulation figures. If in those letters nurses tell the journal what they actually want, then over time this will begin to shape the publishing agenda and ultimately the research one as well. Our experience of letters to journals is that this very seldom happens.

Fifthly, the selection of research topics must be linked to actual research need. Who is best at describing this if not those who do the actual work? Nurses have to take part in local discussions about strategic planning, clinical decision-making and service configuration. They need to know what others are thinking and be politically aware as well as clinically so. They need to make a contribution to these discussions so that their professional opinions are heard, then talk about them to each other at a clinical level to ensure that there is debate about change and development. They need to be supported by their clinical leaders and managers and to do this they have to communicate what it is that they want to achieve. This does not mean that they simply table a shopping list but learn to construct reasoned arguments, backed up by evidence that clearly identifies the necessity to undertake certain courses of action. Part of that action will be the research topics necessary to make appropriate changes. They also need to work with multidisciplinary colleagues to ensure that the aspirations of nurses are not in conflict with others, and, if they are, to find a way of combining the efforts so that different levels of outcomes can be achieved. Researchers who work outside the clinical situation should be invited to development meetings so that they can get a flavour of the discussion. Follow-up meetings with individuals or groups then bring about clarification of the topics and the researcher and practitioners can work together as a team to develop the research project or programme.

Lastly, nurses *must take part in the research work* of others. Whilst this is not necessarily part of the selection process, it is still a method of ensuring that nurses own the research in some way, get used to making decisions about research activities and are better equipped at a later stage to inform others about their requirements of the research process.

2. The quality of nursing research

Much of what we have discussed above relates also to the quality agenda. However, ensuring that the research of others is carried out to an acceptable standard when you are not researching yourself can be fraught with difficulties, not least that the researcher might accuse you of not understanding what it is he or she is trying to achieve. So, the first thing that readers of research must do is *equip themselves with a suitable critiquing tool*, like those used within this book. The use of that tool has to be practised. You cannot expect to be expert at finding the hidden meanings within papers at the first attempt, though it has to be said that surprising results can be achieved very quickly. It is also important that you try to undertake critiques with others, either a friend or a colleague in the clinical area. Discuss each section and compare notes. Gradually your separate reliability measures with that tool will improve and you can begin to use it more often on your own.

Quality in research can mean different things to different people. We understand it to be that the correct research method was used, that the right sample was selected, the data was collected in line with the excepted practice of the method, that data was analysed using appropriate valid measures and the results made sense. Hidden within these few statements, however, are any number of different possibilities, and these can often only be teased out by a careful unpicking of the work. For example, a project was undertaken which explored the application of Parse's theory of human becoming to an in-patient psychiatric setting in the USA (Northrup and Cody, 1998). The method used, descriptive evaluation, was appropriate, whilst the data gathering methods too were sound. Data was analysed and recommendations made in relation to the successful implementation of the theory within the clinical setting. On the face of it this was an interesting and robust piece of research with relevance to P/MH nursing practice. However, careful scrutiny of the paper reveals that the implementation of the theory and the subsequent pre-, mid- and post-data gathering sections were carried out over such a small period of time that genuine implementation simply could not have taken place (Jackson *et al.*, 1999a,b). Therefore the recommendations, which initially had seemed perfectly acceptable, were in fact misleading. While the research was robust, the researched phenomenon was not. Consequently, the recommendations were invalid. Had nurses attempted to implement this work themselves based upon those recommendations they might well have become very disillusioned with their own performance had it not matched their expectations, and valuable time and effort could have been wasted. Establishing *the truth behind research reporting* is at the heart of quality controlling research itself.

One final comment concerning the critiquing process. It is often far easier to find fault with the work of others than to find the good in it. Just because one aspect of a project is suspect does not mean that lessons cannot be learnt from it or that other aspects that are perfectly reliable and valid cannot be considered as useful. *Critiquing does not mean being hypercritical.* It is a balanced process of establishing what is good and what is not, learning from the mistakes and using the successes. All this can occur in a single paper.

3. Reporting and disseminating research

If nurse researchers in the future are to continue to improve upon the effectiveness of their report writing and dissemination activities, those who are the audience for these must read and listen carefully to what is being said and feed back their responses. All scientific journals, and many professional ones, provide a contact address for the lead author of a paper. It is there to enable people to contact them, yet all too often this never happens. If researchers have taken the time to write, it is the responsibility of the reader to report back what they thought of the work, be it critical or complimentary.

Similarly, it would be unfair to expect potential readerships to read everything that is written, so the following represent the basics of a *reading strategy* that combines quality with coverage.

- Choose journals that publish papers that fit your areas of interest or practice; only read those ones and do not read any others unless a particular paper is recommended.
- Speak with your local librarian about finding papers for you on specific topics and requesting searches to be carried out at regular intervals.
- Identify the journals that you and your colleagues or a team have access to, either in the library or through personal subscriptions, and allocate responsibility to each person for reading different journals. Report back to each other on a regular basis those of interest and those requiring specific attention, for whatever reason.
- Keep a reference record of those papers that were relevant to your needs, gradually building up a catalogue you can refer back to at a later date. Try to avoid reading and discarding. There is nothing worse than being unable to

find a paper that you know has the answer you seek. It is almost worse than never having read it in the first place!

■ Use a noticeboard in the clinical area to display copies of new and relevant material.

■ Talk to your colleagues about what you find.

■ Organise a journal club in your ward, unit or team and try to ensure that it has a multidisciplinary attendance.

■ Don't restrict yourself to nursing journals alone.

■ Learn how to quickly decide what should be read now, what can wait till later and what needs to be discarded straight away. It will save you valuable time.

■ Allocate yourself regular periods of quiet time when you can read.

■ Always make notes whilst reading, and attach these to the paper or place them in the journal when you have finished.

■ Check the references used by the author in relevant papers, find them at the library or request them from the librarian. They will enhance your understanding of the paper and the subject matter.

4/5. The practical application of research and research feedback

We have chosen to combine these two sections because, in reality, for the non-researcher, they constitute similar processes. We have already addressed many ways that readers can report back to writers about their thoughts on a paper, but feedback is not just about a person's reaction to a paper. Consider one last very important strategy. The main objective of writing up research for publication has to be that someone will read the work and be inspired enough to want to use what they found within their own practice (Hanily, 1995). *Practice development* is no easy activity and requires careful planning and supervision (Cavanagh and Tross, 1996). If research has been carried out in a robust way, so too must the practice development that implements it into practice. Seeking the advice and opinion from the researcher may be one way of ensuring continuity between the two activities. Even if this is not plausible, nurses using the work of others to enlighten their practice ought to write to the original authors before they begin their development work, informing them of their intentions at intervals during the implementation phases and again once the work is finished and evaluated. Positive feedback of this type does wonders for the researcher's confidence and gives far more meaning to their own work. It might just be the incentive they need to carry on with their endeavours. Of course, once the development work has been carried out – and this may take several years – it too will need to be written up for public consumption; so the cycle of publishing feedback continues, as indeed it should do if we are to progress our knowledge.

Concluding remarks

The reporting and adoption into clinical services and practice of research have to be seen as a joint effort between those who undertake it and those who use it. Increasingly within psychiatric and mental health nursing these two groups are not mutually exclusive, with more and more practitioners carrying out their own investigation. The apparent rift between the two groups is slowly closing, and to a certain degree the aspirations of both groups are common ground. The activities of critical thinking and enquiry are not simply the domain of researchers, just as the processes of clinical decision making and service delivery are not exclusive to practitioners. For mental health nurses to build on their obvious successes to date these facts have to be recognised by all and research has to become an active component in the professional lives of all those whose aim to deliver quality mental health care. As we have shown above, being active in research does not necessarily mean that you are undertaking the work itself, but likewise being a researcher should never mean that your research is not driven by the demands of the practice environment.

Nurse researchers have to embrace all aspects of the nursing agenda, from the so-called soft activities of philosophical and phenomenological enquiry to those of the (equally incorrectly titled) hard research of randomised controlled trials and meta-analysis. In reality they are all part of the same family – simply different methods chosen to suit the form of investigation required and the subject content to which they will be applied. Research methods exist on a sliding scale, a continuum of possibilities that researchers and practitioners alike select as being appropriate to their needs. Whether we are predominantly qualitative or quantitative is immaterial to the main aim of producing a theoretical basis for psychiatric and mental health nursing that is sound, scientific and applicable. Future discipline-specific research will have to show that it meets all these requirements if it is to converge with the demands of an ever more critical professional audience.

Embarking upon research programmes that are exclusively nursing is one goal of nurse-researchers, but there has also to be a commitment to the multidisciplinary research agenda as well. Increasingly nurse-researchers are becoming more sophisticated in their methodological knowledge and their contribution to the wider activity of 'whole community' enquiry is imperative to the successful outcomes of such work. Psychiatric research needs nurses just as much as psychiatric services. The two are interwoven, and research that attempts to exclude one or more of the other parties is bad science, and even worse politics.

Non-researchers also have a responsibility to make their contribution to the research process, albeit in different ways from the researcher. We have shown throughout this book that critically reviewing research is an essential ingredient of the research process itself. The selection of appropriate research topics, the evaluation of the outcomes of that endeavour and the competent application of them into clinical practice and/or professional thinking are all the domain of the non-researcher. Ultimately, being research/evidence-aware must be a guiding factor in the work of all those who aspire to delivering effective care and treatment to those who suffer the debilitating, soul-destroying effects of mental ill health.

References

Akhtar, S. and Samuel, S. (1996) The concept of identity: developmental origins, phenomenology, clinical relevance, and measurement. *Harvard Review of Psychiatry*, **3**, 254–67.

Allen, J. (1998) A survey of psychiatric nurses' opinions of advanced practice roles in psychiatric nursing. *Journal of Psychiatric and Mental Health Nursing*, **5**, 451–62.

Alty, A. (1997) Nurses' learning experience and expressed opinions regarding seclusion practice within one NHS trust. *Journal of Advanced Nursing*, **25**, 786–93.

Ashmore, R. and Carver, N. (2000) Clinical supervision in mental health nursing courses. *British Journal of Nursing*, **9**, 171–6.

Atkinson, M. M. (1996) Psychiatric clinical nurse specialists as intensive case managers for the seriously mentally ill. *Seminars in Nurse Management*, **4**, 130–6.

Barker, P. and Cutcliffe, J. R. (1999) Clinical risk: a need for engagement not observation. *Mental Health Practice*, **2**(8), 8–12.

Barker, P. (1999) Therapeutic nursing for the person in depression. In: *Advanced Practice in Mental Health Nursing* (eds. M. Clinton and S. Nelson), pp. 137–57. Blackwell Science, Oxford.

Barker, P., Jackson, S. and Stevenson, C. (1999) What are psychiatric nurses needed for? Developing a theory of essential nursing practice. *Journal of Psychiatric and Mental Health Nursing*, **6**, 273–82.

Bekker, H., Thornton, J., Airey, C., Connelly, J., Hewison, J., Robinson, M., Lilleyman, J., MacIntosh, M., Maule, A., Michie, S. and Pearman, A. (1999) Informed decision making: an annotated bibliography and systematic review. *Health Technology Assessment*, **3**, 1–156.

Bennett, J., Done, J. and Hunt, B. (1995) Assessing the side-effects of antipsychotic drugs: a survey of CPN practice. *Journal of Psychiatric and Mental Health Nursing*, **2**, 177–82.

Bowers, L., Gournay, K. and Duffy, D. (2000) Suicide and self-harm in inpatient psychiatric units: a national survey of observation policies. *Journal of Advanced Nursing*, **32**, 437–44.

Bowers, L., Jarrett, M., Clark, N., Kiyimba, F. and McFarlane, L. (2000) Determinants of absconding by patients on acute psychiatric wards. *Journal of Advanced Nursing*, **32**, 644–9.

Burnard, P. and Hannigan, B. (2000) Qualitative and quantitative approaches in mental health nursing: moving the debate forward. *Journal of Psychiatric and Mental Health Nursing*, **7**, 1–6.

Butterworth, T. (1991) Generating research in mental health nursing. *International Journal of Nursing Studies*, **28**, 237–46.

Carlsson, G., Dahlberg, K. and Drew, N. (2000) Encountering violence and aggression in mental health nursing: a phenomenological study of tacit caring knowledge. *Issues in Mental Health Nursing*, **21**, 533–45.

Carpenter, M. A. (1991) The process of ethical decision making in psychiatric nursing practice. *Issues in Mental Health Nursing*, **12**, 179–91.

Cavanagh, S. J. and Tross, G. (1996) Utilising research findings in nursing policy and practice: considerations. *Journal of Advanced Nursing*, **24**, 1083–8.

Chien, W. T. (1999) The use of physical restraints to psychogeriatric patients in Hong Kong. *Issues in Mental Health Nursing*, **20**, 571–86.

Chiu, L. (1999) Psychiatric liaison nursing in Taiwan. *Clinical Nurse Specialist*, **13**, 311–14.

Cleary, M., Jordan, R., Horsfall, J., Mazoudier, P. and Delaney, J. (1999) Suicidal patients and special observation. *Journal of Psychiatric and Mental Health Nursing*, **6**, 461–7.

Coffey, M. and Coleman, M. (2001) The relationship between support and stress in forensic community mental health nursing. *Journal of Advanced Nursing*, **34**, 397–407.

Cole, B. V., Scoville, M. and Flynn, L. T. (1996) Psychiatric advance practice nurses collaborate with certified nurse midwives in providing health care for pregnant women with histories of abuse. *Archives of Psychiatric Nursing*, **10**(4), 229–34.

Conrad, B. S. (1998) Maternal depression symptoms and homeless children's mental health risk: Risk and resiliency. *Archives of Psychiatric Nursing* **12**, 50–8.

Croom, S., Procter, S. and Couteur, A. L. (2000) Developing a concept analysis of control for use in child and adolescent mental health nursing. *Journal of Advanced Nursing*, **31**, 1324–32.

Crowe, M. (1998) Developing advanced mental health nursing practice: a process of change. *Australia and New Zealnd Journal of Mental Health Nursing*, **7**, 86–94.

Cutcliffe, J. R. and Goward, P. (2000) Mental health nurses and qualitative research methods: a mutual attraction? *Journal of Advanced Nursing*, **31**, 590–8.

Cutcliffe, J. R. and Hyrkas, K. (2006) Multidisciplinary attitudinal positions regarding clinical supervision. *Journal of Nursing Management*, **14**, 1–11.

Cutcliffe, J. R. and McKenna, H. (2000a) Generic health care workers: the nemesis of psychiatric/mental health nursing? Part one *Mental Health Practice*, **3**(9), 10–14.

Cutcliffe, J. R. and McKenna, H. (2000b) Generic health care workers: the nemesis of psychiatric/mental health nursing? Part two. *Mental Health Practice*, **3**(10), 20–3.

Cutcliffe, J. R. and McKenna, H. P. (2006) Generic nurses: the nemesis of psychiatric/mental health nursing? In: *Key Debates in Psychiatric/Mental Health Nursing* (eds. J. R. Cutcliffe and M. W. Ward), pp. 92–106. Elsevier, Edinburgh.

Cutcliffe, J. R. and Proctor, B. (1998a) An alternative training approach in clinical supervision. Part one. *British Journal of Nursing*, **7**(5), 280–5.

Cutcliffe, J. R. and Proctor, B. (1998b) An alternative training approach in clinical supervision. Part two. *British Journal of Nursing*, **7**(6), 344–50.

Cutcliffe, J. R., Epling, M., Cassedy, P., McGregor, J., Plant, N. and Butterworth, T. (1998a) Ethical dilemmas in clinical supervision: the need for guidelines. *British Journal of Nursing*, **7**(15), 920–3.

Cutcliffe, J. R., Epling, M., Cassedy, P., McGregor, J., Plant, N. and Butterworth, T. (1998b) Ethical dilemmas in clinical supervision: the need for guidelines. *British Journal of Nursing*, **7**(16), 978–82.

Cutcliffe, J., Jackson, A., Ward, M. F., Cannon, B. and Titchen, A. (1998c) Practice development in mental health nursing: Part one. *Mental Health Practice*, **2**, 27–31.

Edwards, D., Burnard, P., Coyle, D., Fothergill, A. and Hannigan, B. (2000) Stress and burnout in community mental health nursing: a review of the literature. *Journal of Psychiatric and Mental Health Nursing*, **7**, 7–14.

Forchuk, C., Jewell, J., Schofield, R., Sircelj, M. and Valledor, T. (1998) From hospital to community: bridging therapeutic relationships. *Journal of Psychiatric and Mental Health Nursing*, **5**, 197–202.

Gournay, K. and Beadsmoore, A. (1995) The report of the clinical standard advisory group: standards of care for people with schizophrenia in the UK and implications for mental health nursing. *Journal of Psychiatric and Mental Health Nursing*, **2**, 359–64.

Gournay, K. and Bowers, L. (2000) Suicide and self harm in in-patient psychiatric units: a study of nursing issues in 31 cases. *Journal of Advanced Nursing*, **32**, 124–31.

Gournay, K., Denford, L., Parr, A. M. and Newell, R. (2000) British nurses in behavioural psychotherapy: a 25-year follow-up. *Journal of Advanced Nursing*, **32**, 343–51.

Gournay, K., Gray, R., Wright, S. and Thornicroft, G. (1997) *Mental Health Nursing in Inpatient Care: a Review of Literature and an Overview of Current Service Provision*. Institute of Psychiatry, London.

Gournay, K., Plummer, S. and Grey, R. (2001) The dream team at the Institute. *Mental Health Practice*, **4**, 15–17.

Gournay, K., Veale, D. and Walburn, J. (1997) Body dysmorphic disorder: pilot randomised controlled trial of treatment implications for nurse therapy research and practice. *Clinical Effectiveness in Nursing*, **1**, 38–46.

Gray, R. and Gournay, K. (2000) What can we do about acute extrapyramidal symptoms? *Journal of Psychiatric and Mental Health Nursing*, **7**, 205–11.

Hanily, F. (1995) A new approach to practice development in mental health. *Nursing Times*, **91**, 34–5.

Hardcastle, M. (1999) Assessment of mental health nursing competence using level III academic marking criteria: the Eastbourne assessment of practice scale. *Nurse Education Today*, **19**, 89–92.

Hazelton, M. (1999) Psychiatric personnel, risk management and the new institutionalism. *Nursing Inquiry*, **6**, 224–30.

International Society of Psychiatric-Mental Health Nurses (1999) *A Position on the Rights of Children in Treatment Settings*. International Society of Psychiatric-Mental Health Nurses, Philadelphia.

Jackson, A., Ward, M. F., Cutcliffe, J., Titchen, A. and Canon, B. (1999a) Practice development in mental health nursing: Part two. *Mental Health Practice*, **2**(5), 20–5.

Jackson, A., Cutcliffe, J., Ward, M., Titchen, A. and Canon, B. (1999b) Practice development in mental health nursing: Part three. *Mental Health Practice*, **2**(7), 24–30.

Jones, J., Lowe, T. and Ward, M. (2000) Inpatient's experiences of nursing observation on an acute psychiatric unit: a pilot study. *Mental Health Care*, **4**, 125–9.

Jones, J., Ward, M., Wellman, N., Hall, J. and Lowe, T. (2000) Psychiatric inpatients' experience of nursing observation: a United Kingdom perspective. *Journal of Psychosocial Nursing and Mental Health Services*, **38**, 10–20.

Kaas, M. J., Dehn, D., Dahl, D., Frank, K., Markley, J. and Hebert, P. (2000) A view of prescriptive practice collaboration: perspectives of psychiatric-mental health clinical nurse specialists and psychiatrists. *Archives of Psychiatric Nursing*, **14**, 222–34.

Kempster, M. (1998) Evidence-based medicine in mental health. *Evidence-Based Nursing*, **1**, 40.

Lakeman, R. (1999) Advanced nursing practice: experience, education and something else. *Nursing Praxis in New Zealand*, **14**, 4–12.

Lutzen, K. and Nordin, C. (1994) Modifying autonomy – a concept grounded in nurses' experiences of moral decision-making in psychiatric practice. *Journal of Medical Ethics*, **20**, 101–7.

Lutzen, K. and Nordin, C. (1995) The influence of gender, education and experience on moral sensitivity in psychiatric nursing: a pilot study. *Nursing Ethics*, **2**, 41–9.

Marks, I. (1977) Costs and benefits of behavioural psychotherapy: a pilot study of neurotics treated by nurse-therapists. *Psychological Medicine*, **7**, 685–700.

Mason, T. (1997) An ethnomethodological analysis of the use of seclusion. *Journal of Advanced Nursing*, **26**, 780–9.

McCabe, S. (2000) Bringing psychiatric nursing into the twenty-first century. *Archives of Psychiatric Nursing*, **14**, 109–16.

McDonald, A. and Gallon, I. (2006) Issues and concerns about 'control and restraint' training: moving the debate forward. In: *Key Debates in Psychiatric/Mental Health Nursing* (eds. J. R. Cutcliffe and M. W. Ward), pp. 181–94. Elsevier, Edinburgh.

McGleish, A. (1996) Leadership in practice: developing leadership in forensic mental health nursing. *Nursing Standard*, **10**, 14–15.

Murrells, T. and Robinson, S. (1997) Developing the nursing contribution to the management of the mental health services. *Journal of Nursing Management*, **5**, 325–32.

Narayan, S. M. and Corcoran, S. (1997) Line of reasoning as a representative of nurses' clinical decision making. *Research in Nursing and Health*, 20, 353–64.

Neilson, P. and Brennan, W. (2001) The use of special observations: an audit within a psychiatric unit. *Journal of Psychiatric and Mental Health Nursing*, **8**, 147–55.

Newell, R. and Gournay, K. (1994) British nurses in behavioural psychotherapy: a 20 year follow-up study. *Journal of Advanced Nursing*, **20**, 53–60.

Noak, J., Conway, S. and Carthy, J. (2006) Managing violence – a contemporary challenge for psychiatric/mental health nurses: the case for 'control and restraint'. In: *Key Debates in Psychiatric/Mental Health Nursing* (eds. J. R. Cutcliffe and M. W. Ward), pp. 168–80. Elsevier, Edinburgh.

Nolan, P. W., Brown, B. and Crawford, P. (1998) Fruits without labour: the implications of Friedrich Nietzsche's ideas for the caring professions. *Journal of Advanced Nursing*, **28**, 251–9.

Northrup, D. T. and Cody, W. K. (1998) Evaluation of the human becoming theory in practice in an acute care psychiatric setting. *Nursing Science Quarterly*, **11**, 23–30.

Onyett, S., Pillinger, T. and Muijen, M. (1995) *Making Community Mental Health Teams Work.* The Sainsbury Centre for Mental Health, London.

Prior, C., Clements, J., Rowett, M., Taylor, D., Rowsell, R. *et al.* (2001) Atypical antipsychotics in the treatment of schizophrenia. *British Medical Journal*, **322**, 924.

Raven, J. and Rix, P. (1999) Managing the unmanageable: risk assessment and risk management in contemporary professional practice. *Journal of Nursing Management*, **7**, 201–6.

Reilly, D. (2001) Obsessive compulsive disorder: cognitive behavioural interventions and the role of the nurse. *Mental Health Practice*, **4**, 16–19.

Ricard, N. (1999) The new challenges of mental health nursing research and practice. *Canadian Journal of Nursing Research*, **31**, 3–15.

Rodriguez, O., Lessinger, J. and Guarnaccia, P. (1992) The societal and organizational contexts of culturally sensitive mental health services: findings from an evaluation of bilingual/bicultural psychiatric programs. *Journal of Mental Health Administration*, **19**, 213–23.

Rogers, E. S., Chamberlin, J., Ellison, M. L. and Crean, T. (1997) A consumer-constructed scale to measure empowerment among users of mental health services. *Psychiatric Services*, **48**, 1042–7.

Sainsbury Centre for Mental Health (1997) Pulling Together: the Future Roles and Training of Mental Health Staff. The Sainsbury Centre for Mental Health, London.

Stordeur, S., Vandenberghe, C. and D'hoore, W. (2000) Leadership styles across hierarchical levels in nursing departments. *Nursing Research*, **49**, 37–43.

Takeuchi, D. T. and Cheung, M. K. (1998) Coercive and voluntary referrals: how ethnic minority adults get into mental health treatment. *Ethnic Health*, **3**, 149–58.

Tang, W. K., Chiu, H., Woo, J., Hjelm, M. and Hui, E. (2001) Telepsychiatry in psychogeriatric service: a pilot study. *International Journal of Geriatric Psychiatry*, **16**, 88–93.

Valimaki, M., Leino-Kilpi, H. and Helenius, H. (1996) Self-determination in clinical practice: the psychiatric patient's point of view. *Nursing Ethics*, **3**, 329–44.

Waddell, C. (2001) So much research evidence, so little dissemination and uptake. *Evidence-Based Mental Health*, **4**, 3–5.

Walters, K. (1990) Critical thinking, rationality and the Vulcanization of students. *Journal of Higher Education*, **61**, 448–67.

Ward, M. F. and Jones, M. (1997) Evaluating the impact of in-patient bed reduction and community nurse increases in one English Mental Healthcare Trust. *Journal of Advanced Nursing*, **26**, 937–45.

Ward, M. W. and Jones, J. (2006) Close observations: the scapegoat of mental health care? In: *Key Debates in Psychiatric/Mental Health Nursing* (eds. J. R. Cutcliffe and M. W. Ward), pp. 257–71. Elsevier, Edinburgh.

Ward, M. F., Titchen, A., Morrell, C., McCormack, B. and Kitson, A. (1998) Using a supervisory framework to support and evaluate a multiproject practice development programme. *Journal of Clinical Nursing*, **7**, 29–36.

Ward, M. F., Armstrong, C., Lelliott, P. and Davies, M. (1999a) Training, skills and caseloads of community mental health support workers involved in case management: evaluation from the initial UK demonstration sites. *Journal of Psychiatric and Mental Health Nursing*, **6**, 187–97.

Ward, M. F., Cutcliffe, J. and Gournay, K. (1999b) A *Review of Research and Practice Development Undertaken by Nurses, Midwives and Health Visitors to Support People with Mental Health Problems*. United Kingdom Central Council for Nurses, Midwives and Health Visitors, London.

Ward, M. F., Jones, J., Gorton, S. and Reed, J. (1999c) The future of mental health nursing. *Nursing Times*, **95**, 51–4.

Ward, M. F., Cutcliffe, J. and Gournay, K. (2000) *The Nursing, Midwifery and Health Visiting Contribution to the Continuing Care of People with Mental Health Problems: A Review and UKCC Action Plan*. United Kingdom Central Council for Nursing, Midwifery and Health Visiting, London.

White, E. (April 1998) Methodological issues in national census research: the case of community mental health nursing in the UK. *Leading Edge: International Nursing Research Conference*, Edinburgh.

White, E. and Brooker, C. (2001) The fourth quinquennial national community mental health nursing census of England and Wales. *International Journal of Nursing Studies*, **38**, 61–70.

Wilkinson, G. (1992) The role of the practice nurse in the management of depression. *International Review of Psychiatry*, **4**, 311–15.

Wooff, K., Goldberg, D. P. and Fryers, T. (1988) The practice of community psychiatric nursing and mental health social work in Salford. Some implications for community care. *British Journal of Psychiatry*, **152**, 783–92.

Younge, O. and Boschma, G. (2006) Debating the integration of psychiatric/mental health nursing content in undergraduate nursing programmes. In: *Key Debates in Psychiatric/Mental Health Nursing* (eds. J. R. Cutcliffe and M. W. Ward), pp. 107–118. Elsevier, Edinburgh.

CHAPTER 15

Evidence-based mental health practice in Europe

Very often Europe is thought of and referred to (by some) as if it were simply a random collection of relatively similar countries, with similar histories, ideals and philosophies. Nothing could be further from the truth. Currently there are 25 countries in the European Union; essentially a federation that includes Finland in its frozen north down to Malta, a small Mediterranean republic, in its hot south; Ireland bordering its west coast and the Czech Republic its eastern face. Add to this 15 other countries, including destinations such as Turkey and Russia, outside the EU but bordering on it, and a further 14 attributed to the WHO region, giving a total of 54, all with with their own histories, alliances, politics and ambitions. Mix in as many as 40 national languages with hundreds of different regional dialects and you begin to realise that 'Europe', apart from being something of a geography teacher's assault course, is really something much larger than the sum of its parts.

Getting people to agree, or even debate, across those borders, whether about territorial issues, who should have which EU operational office in their national capital or just the price of butter, is a process fraught with tension and potential disappointment. As evidence one should be mindful of the 2005 failure to adopt the much vaunted EU-wide constitution following lukewarm acceptance in some member states, rejoicing in others but total rejection by French and Dutch voters as a classic example of how elusive European consensus can be. At least the constitution had an active driving force from parliamentarians committed to international collaboration behind it. As we shall see, something that is more neutral, such as the evidence from critiqued research, has to rely on a far more insidious development to achieve its adoption across national borders.

To chart the progress of something as complex as Evidence-Based Mental Health (EBMH) care throughout the whole of this massive region, with any number of health provider communities, differing care philosophies, resources and expectations, is both beyond the scope of this book. This chapter, therefore, discusses the growth of European EBMH care from an observational standpoint, rather than a catalogue of events. It is more important to explore the problems that this region's different sub-groups have experienced so that we can consider the nature of critiqued evidence more pragmatically from a European standpoint. In so doing, it may then become easier during the critiquing process to appreciate the context in which material has been generated and therefore apportion quality variables to it that more accurately reflect its origin.

There is a further issue to consider, that of national allegiance. Most practitioners will be familiar with the published material emanating from their research and/or educational institutions. Recognising that 'theirs' is not the only way of doing things and that there are other approaches which deliver similar if not necessarily identical clinical outcomes can come as quite a shock to the unprepared. What is worse is that it may also generate academic rejection. This can be loosely defined as a fervent denial of anything that is not written in your national language or published within your native boundaries. While there are obvious difficulties associated with using papers and published material from other countries, not taking account of these during critiquing activities could conceivably be far more problematic in the long run. Meeting mental health specialists from different countries soon awakens you to the realisation that, metaphorically speaking, *the wheel* has been invented in several places, using sometimes similar and sometimes different materials and with differing effects.

Learning across borders is not only professionally illuminating but often refreshingly advantageous. Counteracting the negative effects of academic rejection has potential for a more enlightened workforce but, perhaps more significantly it provides individual practitioners with critiquing options that are not immediately obvious from a uni-national perspective. No one country, no matter how well developed and sophisticated, has all the answers to all the problems. Similarly, no one set of mental health practitioners currently has all the material it needs from its own researchers to be able to answer all the questions posed. Any suggestion that it does is equally both short-sighted and arrogant. Solving similar problems, but from different national perspectives, allows the practitioner to explore the differences in practice that provide the bedrock of professional strength rather than simply congratulating themselves on the similarities – a stance that will ultimately lead to clinical stagnation. What mental health care needs is choice and alternatives if its knowledge base is to progress, and this patently cannot come from a uni-national reliance on internal and culturally bound agendas.

Understanding how EBMH care has developed within the European context is therefore important for a variety of reasons but chief amongst them is the fact that opening the academic borders to focus on material stemming from outside the accepted *national norm* increases the potential for effective problem solving.

National boundaries and politics

To fully appreciate the development of European EBMH care one needs to consider Europe from historical and geographical perspectives. There have always
been certain alliances that, to this day, bind individual counties with neighbours
and other politically sympathetic states. Those politics exert influence throughout the whole of the national infrastructure as well as across borders. Their
subsequent influence over the nature of research, health care and specifically
mental health care, cannot be over stressed here. Without a doubt health care is
a major political topic. The ways in which health care is resourced, supported,
funded and delivered are all matters of the gravest concern to governments,
because along with other services, such as education and social services, their
performance is a reflection of governmental efficiency. Because these services
are directly linked to the aspirations of their populations they have to be presented in a positive light and as meeting the needs of the country.

Imagine a situation where the researchers of one country discover that a much
heralded approach to the care of people with so-called 'personality disorders'
adopted in a member state actually has harmful effects that outweigh its clinical
efficacy. Consider the dilemma of a government that has invested millions in
such things as a building program to support the housing of the approach for its
growing population of diagnosed personality disordered people, the educational
and training programs for those who see this work as a career development, and
the publicity campaigns designed to show the general population that their government is both cognisant of their needs and making society safer. Imagine, too,
the crisis in confidence for internal researchers who had brokered the approach
in the first place. What are both these sections of the community to do with these
new potentially aggressive findings? This is a rhetorical question that if posed
would need to be considered against the backdrop of Europe's recent devolu-
tional history. However, if it were to be answered it would need to address certain key factors, namely the period in history, the political allegiances, cultural
anomalies and, increasingly, the influence of languages.

Europe can be divided into several regions, but from the point view of establishing a history of the growth of EBMH care there are probably two major
ones and six smaller (relatively speaking) ones. These are categorised by their
relationships with other countries, their history, their geographical location, the
power they exert within the medical community, and their primary language.

The two main regions are predominantly those that are within the European
Union and those that are not. This last can be broken down to those that border
the existing EU member states and those that are more distant from them. Interestingly, the further away from central Europe that you progress within this
region the more dominant are factors that militate the sharing of knowledge
because of the absence of an international communication infrastructure. These

countries, and to a certain degree the second region as a whole, also share one other key element, that of a fundamentally different philosophical view from the other regions about the nature, causation and treatment of mental health problems (or psychiatric illnesses) generally.

The sub-regions of the first group can be identified as the Nordic countries, central and western Europe, French-speaking nations, German-speaking nations, the Iberian and Mediterranean countries and eastern Europe, including the Balkan states. Through proximity alone it can be seen that these countries share several key elements in the ability to communicate across borders and therefore develop interrelated research activities. It is from these common research programs that the growth of evidence has emerged, but rather than being a Europe-wide phenomenon, it has been traditionally a regional or sub-regional one. Countries with common or related languages, political dimensions, borders and philosophical values are more likely to be accepting of research material from within these separate enclaves. While this may be good from the point of view of at least some sharing of ideas for the development of mental health care it does still mean that the public face of these services will be dramatically different across the different regions, with potentially one providing significantly more effective care for the person with mental health problems (for some the mentally ill) then others.

Indeed, the situation is further complicated by the fact that even the regions themselves do not exist within a research vacuum. Europe is to a greater or lesser degree influenced by the work of practitioners and investigators in the North American communities, Australasia and increasingly South America and Japan. Considering that the evidence-based medicine movement as we know it today originated in the North American health care and academic environment, it might be significant that if one traces the development of EBMH care in Europe one finds that the closer countries and/or regions are to sharing ideas with this national region the more advanced are their systems for implementing evidence-based care. And it also has to be said that if one were to look at a picture of Europe's evidence-based activities prior to the national changes that have taken place there in the last 15 years, one would get a totally different view of things. The allegiances within the Eastern Bloc countries, predominantly influenced by the psychiatric activities of the old USSR, made for a region in its own right and one which seldom had a great deal in common with the rest of the wider professional community. As we shall see, this situation has changed dramatically and most of those countries have now become aligned with other regions within the European context, and, notably, within evidence-based mental health care.

It would be wrong to conclude this section without making comment about the growth of the EBMH movement within Europe generally. To a certain degree there have been three regions that have largely followed the direction for this as conceived by McMaster University in Canada: the Nordic, central and western, and German-speaking (mainly Germany, Austria, Luxemburg, Switzerland and some parts of northern Italy and southern Belgium) regions. To a certain extent these have mirrored each other, although, as will be seen, because of language issues much of what has happened in the German-speaking region is unknown to the vast majority of professionals within the other regions.

The other regions have developed in their own way. The Iberian region has had a major influence from Italy, where, two decades ago, for whatever reason, it was decided to close all the major mental health care institutions and deposit their populations into community facilities. The 'experiment' was not an unmitigated failure but it cannot be described as a success either. However, key conclusions derived from this period have gradually filtered into the literature and have influenced thinkers elsewhere – though less so if published in anything other than the English language. Spain, Portugal and now Malta have tended to be led almost entirely by psychiatric, rather than nursing, research and literature.

The Nordic states present a different picture. Contrary to popular belief outside these countries (Sweden, Norway, Denmark, Finland, Iceland, Faroe Islands), they do not all share a common language, though with the exception of Finnish (which is completely different from all the others) they are able to communicate reasonably well on a conversational level. The professional language remains English and this has meant that North American literature and, increasingly over the last 10 years that from the UK, has heavily influenced their thinking. Their own research activities are extremely active and national nursing journals provide an outlet for the published material.

The French region (France, Switzerland, northern Italy, parts of Belgium, Monaco) has developed its evidence base in tune with the North American approach, but very much 'in-house'. The result is that almost no evidence developed within France specifically reaches the wider professional community. The eastern Europe and Balkan states are a separate entity in that they are only just beginning to appreciate the nature of evidence-based activities. Much of the material they have has either been translated into local languages or is essentially medical in nature. The effect, as will be discussed later, is to disenfranchise the nursing or care staff, because either no research has been carried out to support their actions, or the material they do have only suggests courses of actions for their medical colleagues.

The impact of language

One of the main problems associated with evidence-based mental health care is its dependence on the medical model and, subsequently, diagnosis and diagnostic values. This has had a direct bearing on the quality of the evidence and the nature of concurrent EBMH care or psychiatric/mental health nursing. Writing from Switzerland, the Assistant Director of Zurich University Hospital states that there are three fundamental reasons why this dependence has had such a negative influence within psychiatry, namely: the validity of psychiatric diagnosis is limited; the approach cannot track the multiplicity of presentations for psychiatric disorders, therefore devaluing its effects; and the strong focus that evidence-based psychiatry places on decision making does not reflect the reality for psychiatrists or therapists (Maier, 2006). A comprehensive discussion of the arguments for and against these issues falls outside the scope of this chapter and this book, but the authors would like to add a further item. The vast majority of diagnostic values stem from either DSM-IV or ICD-10 and their linguistic derivatives. Yet witnessing the use of different diagnoses across countries shows that there is limited validity to their use and what appears to be schizophrenia in one will be conduct disorder in another; what is bi-polar disorder in one may be multi-infarct dementia in another etc.

Such a situation leads Levine and Fink (2006) to ask: if the diagnosis itself fails to capture the essence of a patient's condition when interpreted by clinicians, how can evidence of that particular condition be used to influence treatment programs? Although countries such as Turkey played a big part in developing DSM-IV, can it really be said that the language transfer does not play a big part in determining the interpretation of the diagnosis as applied to the local context? This then brings into question whether or not larger scale research activities based around systematic reviews and meta-analysis are really accessing information derived from similar sources. Crucially, it should be acknowledged that the critiquing process should be able to determine whether or not the validity of an individual paper warrants its inclusion in a progressive study, but most papers do not ask for evidence of diagnostic criteria, only diagnoses.

Certainly Europe-wide evaluations of mental health/illness burdens are being undertaken, and in the case of Pini *et al.* (2005) across ten different countries – only four of which shared a common language. The review explored studies undertaken in these countries to investigate the impact of bi-polar disorder as categorised in DSM-III-R, DSM-IV and ICD-10. The problem here is that DSM-III was replaced over 10 years ago, yet was still being used in European studies and reviewed in 2004/5. The conclusions from this review were none too startling, but had they been crucial to the delivery of specialist mental health care this might have suggested the provision of inappropriate interventions. This issue is one of languages, though of course the definition and interpretation of the diagnosis is part of this. Understanding within one country may differ from that of another, though the variables at play also include issues of training, support and audit.

One further example of the problems associated with language use may be useful at this juncture. It relates to a pan-European study undertaken in 2004/5 with the express purpose of assessing the quality of European treatment guidelines in the field of mental health produced by national psychiatric associations. The main focus was the question of whether or not the development process of the guidelines followed basic principles of evidence-based medicine (Stiegler, 2005). No fewer than 61 clinical practice guidelines, from 14 different European countries, were evaluated. The documents had all been produced during what could be described as the active evidence-based period, namely 1998–2003. Both the results and the methods are interesting for this chapter. The guidelines were found to be of only reasonable quality in 50% of cases, but more significantly only 50% of them were based upon any form of evidence. The primary languages they were written in were several and the interpretation of what was written was based on both translations and local interpretations. The question arises about the authenticity of the material that was being used, not the quality of the investigative procedures. Gartlehner (2004) suggests that we get around this problem by using databases established in native languages, arguing that it would increase communication between different member states, raise the profile of European evidence-based practice and reduce costs. The authors of this book are yet to be convinced by a strategy that appears to be nothing more than that which already exists, but on a far more formal footing. However, there is some evidence to suggest that this situation may be changing. In a German study, Kilian *et al.* (2003) scientifically evaluated the performance of a German translation of a tool to explore mental health service provision needs. The statistical assessment indicated that it was comparable with the other European versions of the instrument. While this in itself is not conclusive evidence of good practice, it is a least a step in the right direction, but, as this study also shows, the lengths that clinicians have to go through to translate and back translate are very time-consuming.

Obviously the problem of language, or should we say, different languages, is one that will always plague organisations, institutions and countries. The problem for EBMH care is that too few of the personnel who try to access the literature from either different countries or using different languages have either the linguistic skills, or access to them, to be able to make sense of what is happening elsewhere. Additionally, if P/MH nurses in a developing country are trying to access research evidence from other areas this probably means that as a first stop there is little or no material in their own country/language that they can refer to direct. The significance of this is discussed in the next section, but from a linguistic point of view it means that P/MH nurses in this situation are being disenfranchised by a situation over which they have little or no control.

The effect of roles and responsibilities of P/MH nurses

Given that Europe has a total WHO-affiliated country count of 54 it seems unlikely that the roles and responsibilities of those working in these countries with people with mental health problems have similar jobs and responsibilities. In fact, in several of the Eastern European countries, the word *nurse* does not have any real meaning, let alone the term *psychiatric/mental health nurse*. Medical Assistants and Aides are far more likely to be called in to 'care' for the person with mental health problems and the 'care' they offer will be determined very much by the medical officer in charge of the patient's treatment program. In other countries, within both the EU and non-EU regions you will find countries where P/MH nurses hold positions of relative authority, and are well educated and sophisticated practitioners with a high degree of clinical decision making autonomy. If these two poles represent the extremes of practice, then it seems likely that there are any number of variations sitting in between.

There does seem to be a correlation between the roles of nurses, the inter-disciplinary relationship between them and their medical colleagues and the involvement in, and uptake of, evidence development. In countries such as Holland, Belgium, the four countries of the UK and the Nordic region there appears to be a degree of professional autonomy for nurses that is matched by their interest in EBMH care. There are sufficient national and international journals for these practitioners to read and submit their work to and their appreciation of the English language means they can also access the North American and Australasia publications with relative ease. Also, with the possible exception of Holland, where only recently has an advanced practitioner Master's programme started, these countries have active post-graduate and doctoral programmes for nurses. As one of the precursors for these types of programme is a 'healthy appetite' for clinical evidence and the necessity to undertake research, it seems likely that this has also contributed to the obvious interest in EBMH care in these countries.

In the case of the UK these countries also have active evidence-based medical involvement with several world centres being resident there (The Cochrane Initiative, The York Research and Dissemination Centre, various WHO collaborating centres and several evidence-based journals). With nurses having ready access to these resources it is not surprising that the UK has been one of the first to take an active role in its development. Its nurses too have a very firm grasp of their roles and with over 55,000 nurses holding a qualification in psychiatric/mental health care the power of numbers has also predisposed the discipline to make its own decisions about what it does and does not research. There are some problems with this system, because allowing every individual nurse on higher academic courses to choose their own topic to research tends to mean that much work is done that does not fit with any overall research strategy.

However, at least those nurses have a sense of direction and are involved in the research, or research critiquing, process.

For the German-speaking countries the situation is very similar except that nurses there do not have quite the same autonomy, nor do they all have the rather unlimited access to resources that their western, central and Nordic colleagues do. Their numbers are also marginally smaller and medical staff have far more control over the clinical scene. For countries in the other regions the situation becomes less pronounced in favour of EBMH involvement the further they move away from the west. This is also consistent with their dependence on medical decision making, on diagnosis-led treatments and on therapy being delivered by staff other than nurses. This is more marked within the eastern European and Baltic states region, where there is an absence of nurses who can speak or read English, very few nurses with higher academic qualifications and practically no resources at basic clinical level to support and advocate the use of evidence in nursing practice. The one exception to this is Turkey, where there is quite a large cohort of nurses with Master's level qualifications and a few with Doctorates. Unfortunately, with no exceptions, they are all employed in the universities, none being in clinical practice. While this is obviously good for knowledge generation amongst graduate nurses, it also means that practising nurses have limited clinically based role models on whom to base their clinical use of evidence. In addition, Turkish mental health care is dominated by medical decision making. Countries like the Czech Republic and Hungary have similar situations except that they have practically no higher academically trained nurses, added to the fact that evidence is almost totally generated and used by psychiatrists. The nurse's role in these countries is to do as instructed by the medical team and this seems to suggest that with diminished roles and responsibilities, lack of higher education opportunities and medical dominance the possibility of undertaking or even accessing evidence for practice is extremely limited.

One of the key pieces of research undertaken on this subject by European nurses emanated from Finland (Oranta *et al.*, 2002). The researchers attempted to establish the barriers inhibiting the uptake of knowledge by nurses to inform their practice. From a sample of 316 registered nurses they discovered that the main barriers were that most research was published in a foreign language and, significantly, that medical staff would not cooperate with the implementation of evidence even when it was available. This lack of multidisciplinary support for nurses wishing to perhaps influence the clinical setting suggests that medical control has more influence over the management of evidence than many nurses would like to believe. Yet, paradoxically, it is the medical staff who themselves generate much of the evidence that is implemented (Richter and Nollau, 2000).

On a final note for this section, while recognising that the development of EBMH care could have any number of different variables that would affect its progress, it does seem that throughout Europe there is a large body of evidence available if only staff were in a position to access it. The anomaly is that if it is in a foreign language it is not going to be read by other nationals. The tragedy of this situation is that somewhere there could be a piece of research, say in German or Italian, Serbian or Russian, that answers the questions you have been asking, but, sadly, you may never know about it.

Evidence-based mental health developments within the regions

So what type of evidence has been generated within the European regions over the last few years, and specifically since the mid-1990s? Where has the energy of the researchers been focused and who has been responsible for knowledge generation? Three general themes arise: medical treatments (including randomised controlled trials of the new breed of anti-psychotics and anti-depressants, issues relating to the generation of evidence and clinical governance), nursing management/supervision (including the development of skills within a cognitive behavioural framework, special or close observations and forensic engagement), and service standards/provisions (including risk and cost effectiveness). These are centred around certain psychopathological presentations, namely personality disorders, schizophrenia and depression/suicide. Dominating all of these is an overarching interest in patient and carer involvement.

What is interesting is that in the German-speaking countries there is a whole raft of research that will never be made available to those who cannot speak the language. Yet contained within this material are culturally bound studies that mirror those in the professional press of other countries and in other languages. For example, Lang *et al.* (2002) undertook a large study of psychiatric patients' experiences to identify patients with different treatment experiences, evaluating differences in quality of life among those patients, exploring changes in quality of life following community resettlement, and attempting to find predictors of overall life satisfaction. This Austrian paper, and/or elements of it, easily complements studies in the international press such as that in England (Secker *et al.* 2001), Italy (Lasalvia *et al.* 2002) and Slovenia (Svab *et al.* 2002), although there is no evidence of either triangulated or reciprocal referencing. The same can be said for other parts of the professional press, but to a certain degree those of the Nordic, eastern and Baltic states regions tend to attempt to publish significant research findings in either UK- or American-based journals. This is particularly the case in psychiatry and increasingly so within P/MH nursing.

However, if one explores the nursing literature there is a completely different picture, possibly reflecting the progress on nursing professionalism and autonomy. Ryrie *et al.* (1997) considered the roles and responsibilities of the P/MH nurse in a liaison psychiatric service within the accident and emergency department of a large UK general hospital. What is important about this paper from an EBMH care perspective is the emphasis placed upon the autonomy, advanced practice requirements and educational development of the nurses within the team. While accepting that much of the published material on this approach to care was written during the mid-1990s, and accepting the review comments of Callaghan *et al.* (2003) that most of the literature and research comes essentially from either North America or the UK and is produced mainly by psychiatrists, there is evidence of significant non-English publications within this area, and by nurses. Not this time in a German publication, but a French one, Tortonese (2001) explored specifically the roles and responsibilities of nurses within such a team and many of the points raised were similar to those of the earlier UK-based study of Ryrie *et al.* Again, and this time to the detriment of the French study, there was no evidence of cross-referencing and therefore it must be assumed that Tortonese had not accessed the Ryrie *et al.* study while preparing his own research. Oranta *et al.* (2002) pointed to the problems associated with language, but there also seems to be a divide between different regions and the progress their nurses have made in relation to higher academic education and the adoption of advanced clinical roles.

Both the Tortonese and Ryrie *et al.* studies highlight significant autonomy for the nurses involved. Yet, in many of the other regions this autonomy simply does not exist and is reflected in the absence of any research (and consequently published evidence) within professional publications of any nationality or language. Indeed, in approximately half of the 25 countries of the EU there is no national nursing publication and certainly fewer than that have something dedicated to P/MH nursing.

It seems self-evident therefore that where nurses working in mental health care have little of the autonomous roles associated with advanced practice the discipline's general dependence upon their medical colleagues is very high. In a significant editorial comment, Gournay (2001, p. 473) wrote that he feared many of the traditional roles of P/MH nurses (in the UK) would eventually be undertaken by 'generic mental health workers'. It may well be that in many European countries this is already the norm and has been so for most of the history of their psychiatric services. Thus the ability of some groups of national nurses to contribute the growth of European EBMH care is limited. But it is not just the relative position of nursing *vis à vis* their medical colleagues that acts against a general European development of research influencing practice. The report of the Workforce Action Team of the UK National Service Framework (Brooker *et al.*, 2000) discussed the issues of higher educational resourcing to support such a venture. From this document it can be seen that it is not that a country has a university structure that is so important, but that this structure has established within it a firm footing for health care and, within this, a vigorous and active nursing section. Sadly, with few exceptions (possibly Turkey and Estonia), the further east and south one progresses in Europe the less this is the case. P/MH nursing's contribution to the emergent European EBMH care agenda will depend heavily on rectifying the problems identified by Oranta *et al.* (2002) and finding solutions to the discipline's ability to control its own work practices.

In summary

From a European perspective the term 'EBMH care', as an entity, will mean different things to different people depending upon where they live within Europe. The development and gradual evolution of evidence-based practice activities will also depend on certain factors, and once again these may well be influenced by geographical positioning within the discrete regions of Europe. However, there are a series of key indicators as described in this chapter that may determine the successful implementation of evidence to practice irrespective of country of practice and/or origin. Box 15.1 provides an overview of these.

What is clear is that from a mental health perspective, Europe generally lagged behind North America, in part because this was where the approach was first developed, and in part because of significant differences in the philosophy of mental health care provision. What is not so clear is what the future holds. Will we see a gradual shift towards a more even spread of evidence across the different regions, and if so what will precipitate such a growth? There is currently no evidence to suggest that this is likely to happen within the foreseeable future; however, there are some signs that attitudes towards certain of the negative key indicators of Box 15.1 are changing for the better (see, for example, Ruggeri *et al.*, 2004; Leonard, 2004 and Paley *et al.*, 2003).

Whatever the outcome, issues such as what constitutes evidence, where evidence comes from and how it should be used effectively within a clinical situation will continue to dominate both professional and politic debates. However, the ability of P/MH nurses across Europe to be able to critique the product of research and subsequently use critical thinking in their work should not be dependent on whether or not forces outside of the discipline see such activities as being important. For European P/MH nursing to develop it has to establish control over the material that it uses to influence the way it practices and that can only happen by addressing the issues of Box 15.1.

Box 15.1 Issues that either support or oppose the growth of European evidence-based mental health care

For:

- Having common beliefs and values
- Sharing common roles and responsibilities and understanding what they are
- Having access to resources and support for EBMH
- Having nurses with higher degrees working in clinical practice
- Gaining support on a multidisciplinary level
- Linking political strategies to clinical outcomes
- Teaching staff how to undertake research critique

Against:

- Having differing political aspirations from either researchers or publications
- Having very different languages from either researchers or their publications
- Having different interpretations of diagnostic values
- Working with unsupportive medical colleagues
- A lack of roles for nurses
- A lack of higher education opportunities for clinical based nursing staff

---

References

Brooker C., Gournay K., O'Halloran P. and Bailey D. (2000) *Mapping the Capacity of the English University System to Deliver National Service Framework Priorities*. Report to the Workforce Action Team. Department of Health, London.

Callaghan, P., Eales, T. and Bowers, L. (2003)) A review of research on the structure, process and outcome of liaison mental health services. *Journal of Psychiatric and Mental Health Nursing*, **10**(2), 155–65.

Gartlehner, G. (2004) Evidence-based medicine breaking the borders – a working model for the European Union to facilitate evidence-based health care. *Wien Medical Wochenschrift*, **154**, 127–32.

Gournay, K. (2001) Mental health nursing: what happens next? Guest editorial. *Journal of Psychiatric and Mental Health Nursing*, **8**, 473–6.

Kilian, R., Roick, C., Bernert, S., Matschinger, H., Mory, C., Becker, T. and Angermeyer, M. C. (2001) Instruments for the economical evaluation of psychiatric service systems: methodological foundations of the European standardisation and the German adaptation. *Psychiatric Praxis*, **28** (suppl. 2), 74–8.

Lang, A., Steiner, E., Berghofer, G., Henkel, H., Schmitz, M., Schmidl, F. and Rudas, S. (2002) Quality of life and other characteristics of Viennese mental health care users. *International Journal of Social Psychiatry*, **48**, 59–69.

Lasalvia, A., Ruggeri, M. and Santolini, N. (2002) Subjective quality of life: its relationship with clinician-rated and patient-rated psychopathology. The South-Verona Outcome Project 6. *Psychotherapy and Psychosomatics*, **71**(5), 275–84.

Leonard, S. (2004) The development and evaluation of a telepsychiatry service for prisoners. *Journal of Psychiatric and Mental Health Nursing*, **11**(4), 461–8.

Levine, R. and Fink, M. (2006) The case against evidence-based principles in psychiatry. *Medical Hypotheses*, 3 May.

Maier, T. (2006) Evidence-based psychiatry: understanding the limitations of a method. *Journal of Evaluation in Clinical Practice*, **12**, 325–9.

Oranta, O., Routasalo, P. and Hupli, M. (2002) Barriers to and facilitators of research utilization among Finnish registered nurses. *Journal of Clinical Nursing*, **11**, 205–13.

Paley, G., Myers, J., Patrick, S., Reid, E. and Shapiro, D. A. (2003) Practice development in psychological interventions: mental health nurse involvement in the conversational model of psychotherapy. *Journal of Psychiatric and Mental Health Nursing*, **10**(4), 494–8.

Pini, S., de Queiroz, V., Pagnin, D., Pezawas, L., Angst, J., Cassano, G. B. and Wittchen, H. U. (2005) Prevalence and burden of bipolar disorders in European countries. *European Neuropsychopharmacology*, **15**, 425–34.

Richter, R. A. and Nollau, M. (2000) Perspectives of psychiatric care in Leipzig: deinstitutionalization from the viewpoint of neurologist/psychiatrist in private practice and the work of consortium of community psychiatric services. *Psychiatric Praxis*, **27** (suppl. 2), 95–9.

Ruggeri, M., Bisoffi, G., Lasalvia, A., Amaddeo, F., Bonetto, C. and Biggeri, A. (2004) A longitudinal evaluation of two-year outcome in a community-based mental health service using graphical chain models. The South-Verona outcome project 9. *International Journal of Methods in Psychiatric Research*, **13**(1), 10–23.

Ryrie I., Roberts, M. and Taylor, R. (1997) Liaison psychiatric nursing in an inner city accident and emergency department. *Journal of Psychiatric and Mental Health Nursing*, **4**, 131–6.

Secker, J., Gulliver, P., Peck, E., Robinson, J., Bell, R. and Hughes, J. (2001) Evaluation of community mental health services: comparison of a primary care mental health team and an extended day hospital service. *Health and Social Care in the Community*, **9**(6), 495–503.

Stiegler, M., Rummel, C., Wahlbeck, K., Kissling, W. and Leucht, S. (2005) European psychiatric treatment guidelines: is the glass half full or half empty? *European Psychiatry*, **20**, 554–8.

Svab, V., Tomori, M., Zalar, B., Ziherl, S., Dernovsek, M. Z. and Tavcar, R. (2002) Community rehabilitation service for patients with severe psychotic disorders: the Slovene experience. *International Journal of Social Psychiatry*, **48**(2), 156–60.

Tortonese, M. (2001) The nurse in liaison psychiatry... social aspects. *Soins Psychiatrie*, **216**, 44–6.

Key points arising from the examples had we used the NPNR Journal Club approach to critiquing research

Example 1: Parahoo (1999)

1. The study identifies the limited familiarity with and use of research by many psychiatric/mental health nurses, yet it also highlighted the same nurses' enthusiasm to make use of research. Consequently, the need for support/ facilities (of various types) to help these nurses become 'research-based' practitioners is reiterated.
2. Members felt that the differences between 'evidence-based' and 'research-based' practice were not made clear in the paper, and this important difference needed to be highlighted.
3. Members were uncomfortable with the implicit assumption concerning the hegemony of RCTs and felt that it would have been more appropriate to point out that different research methods produce different types of knowledge and are suitable for different research questions, with no one method therefore being 'better' than another.

Example 2: Pullen et al. (1999)

1. Given the wide range of confounding variables and interactions of variables that could impact on patterns of drug/alcohol use, and its alleged relationship with religiosity, it may not be wise to posit such relationships as straightforward 'cause and effect' hypotheses.

2. Given the well-established relationship between drug/alcohol abuse and 'religiosity', the value or purpose of another study to further confirm that which already appears to be known appears to be in question, particularly when many unanswered yet relevant questions within this substantive area remain.

3. While there is an abundance of literature that lends support to the argument of attending to one's 'spiritual' needs and there is evidence that such needs can be met by engaging in 'religious' activities, it would be inaccurate to consider religious activities as the *only* way of meeting such needs.

Example 3: Hannigan (1999)

1. Members stated that the sampling strategy could be regarded as one of the strengths of the paper since it sampled the total population (i.e. each education centre that provided the CPN course). Furthermore, it achieved a response rate of 82%, which is high for a postal return survey. Therefore the members felt that such results could be taken to be indicative or representative of the total population.

2. While the paper included some discussion of the findings, there was a distinct view that perhaps the author had not asked certain 'big' questions within the discussion, and therefore perhaps the study missed an opportunity.

3. Members felt that the apparent honesty of the author, with regard to both the limitations and reporting of the study, could be regarded as one of the strengths of the paper, as this honesty was evident throughout.

Example 4: Fletcher (1999)

1. The paper draws further attention to the potential problems associated with 'custodial' methods of 'constant observations', re-emphasises the difficulties some nurses have with such methods of 'care' and illustrates the potential value of care approaches that focus on engaging such clients. Furthermore, it reiterates that care of the suicidal client is a particularly skilful, yet demanding activity.

2. Consideration must be given to ethical issues in all research, and research with vulnerable groups (e.g. mental health clients) may present particular ethical concerns which must be addressed. Failure to do so can be seen to be undermining the credibility of the research.

3. The paper adds support to the argument that service user feedback/data should be included in studies that are concerned with service evaluation or research.

Example 5: Allen (1998)

1. While the author claimed to have undertaken a qualitative analysis of the comments written in response to the questions, members felt that the author did not appear to have undertaken what could be accurately described as qualitative research. Of particular concern was the author's claim that counting the same word or phrase constituted qualitative data analysis.
2. While the research did not uncover any new insights, the findings did reiterate theoretical (and valuable) positions, in particular the importance in ensuring that advanced nursing roles do not become a 'dumping ground' for practices no longer desired by medics.
3. Members acknowledged that the conclusions were partially justified by the results. However, in the light of the methodological limitations, the possible unrepresentative nature of the sample, the absence of any reliability or validity measures, and the cross-sectional nature of the study, it might have been more appropriate for the author to phrase his conclusion in a tentative manner, rather than the 'assertive' manner used in the paper.

Example 6: Pejlert *et al.* (1998)

1. The structure and arrangement of the information contained in the paper was thought to be somewhat equivocal and confusing.
2. The study raised an important issue that is repeatedly highlighted, in that a study that discusses the opinions or elicits the experiences of recipients of care illustrates that nurses who were kind and understanding were equated with providing good care.
3. The paper contains too much tautological and unnecessary text, and consequently this text may detract from the impact of the overall message of the paper.

Example 8: Veeramah (1995)

1. There is evidence of only limited discussion of the implications for nursing practice/theory/research. Members highlighted that there are many relevant issues relating to this matter and the findings of the research, and felt that the researcher rather 'sold himself/herself short'.
2. The paper does make specific recommendations and these were felt to have sense and value. However, while they appear to have some resonance with the results, they do not appear to have been uncovered through the research process. That is, many of the recommendations do not appear to have evolved directly from the results, and consequently the members felt that some of these had an element of impracticability.
3. The paper was reasonably well written and it appears to have been written purposefully to enable the reader's understanding. (Indeed, the author makes such claims within the paper.) Consequently, one of the strengths of the paper can be considered to be the absence of unnecessary jargon or tautology.

Example 9: Whittington and Wykes (1994)

1. While the paper raises some interesting points and perhaps indicates several possible directions for future research, the model presented and subsequently tested (in part) in the paper was felt to be somewhat simplistic and provided little understanding of the complex interplay of processes, dynamics and variables which appear to be involved in client violence, nurses' behaviours and nurses' feelings.
2. The paper addresses an important substantive issue and was considered to be 'brave' for its willingness to broach potentially awkward and often emotive subjects such as client violence and the nurse's role in perpetuating this violence.
3. The paper contains important implications for psychiatric/mental health nursing practice, yet these were largely implicit in the paper, and perhaps would have benefited from being made explicit and from undergoing a more rigorous discussion.

Index